Oil Pulling Therapy

Detoxifying and Healing the Body Through Oral Cleansing

Dr. Bruce Fife ━━━━━

Piccadilly Books, Ltd.
Colorado Springs, CO

Every effort has been made to ensure that the information contained in this book is complete and accurate. However, neither the publisher nor the author is engaged in rendering professional advice or services to the individual reader. The information contained in this book is not intended as a substitute for consulting with your physician. All matters regarding your health require medical supervision. Neither the author nor the publisher shall be liable or responsible for any loss or damage allegedly arising from any information or suggestion in this book.

Piccadilly Books, Ltd.
P.O. Box 25203
Colorado Springs, CO 80936, USA
www.piccadillybooks.com
info@piccadillybooks.com

Library of Congress Cataloging-in-Publication Data
Fife, Bruce, 1952-
   Oil pulling therapy: detoxifying and healing the body through oral cleansing/ by Bruce Fife.
        p. cm.
   Includes bibliographical references and index.
   ISBN 978-0-941599-67-2
   1. Detoxification (Health) 2. Vegetable oils--Therapeutic use. 3. Mouth--care and hygiene. 4. Oral manifestations of general diseases. I. Title.
   RA784.5.F54 2008
   613--dc22
                                    2008015136

Printed in the USA

Table of Contents

"A new truth is a new sense, for with it comes the ability to see things we could not see before—and things which cannot be seen by those who do not have that new truth."

Weston A. Price, D.D.S.

Chapter 1

A New Approach To Better Health

OIL PULLING GAVE BACK MY LIFE

Take a spoonful of vegetable oil, put it in your mouth, and swish it around? Tara couldn't believe it. How could sucking on oil improve one's health? It just didn't seem to make any sense. But her doubts turned into conviction as she started the unusual therapy.

"I began oil pulling seven months ago," says Tara of Melbourne, Australia, in a posting to www.earthclinic.com. "I suffered with chronic fatigue for 14 years…I was confined to bed rest and had limited mobility."

Chronic fatigue was not her only problem. Tara also suffered from fibromyalgia. "I was in chronic pain and was suicidal," says Tara. "I could barely move my tongue inside my mouth and could not walk. I was so ill; I had never experienced anything like the severity of this before."

Oil pulling dramatically shifted things for her, with noticeable improvement every day. "I kept oil pulling, and changes occurred incrementally every day until after a couple of weeks my health was back to normal…I am now more fit and active, and don't need to rest as much. I had been living this way for years, and oil pulling gave me my life back. It also cleared up a skin problem I had when nothing else seemed to work…Oil pulling has changed my life!" Within just a few short weeks Tara had overcome two chronic illnesses that doctors say cannot be cured.

"This is the most powerful therapy that has ever come to me," says Lee, of West Bountiful, Utah, in a posting to www.earthclinic.com. "I've been oil pulling, and my wife also, for one month and three days. To us it has been overwhelming! Many very effective changes have occurred in our bodies, which allows me to recognize how powerful this therapy is. I have far more peace of mind, extremely improved digestion and elimination, sleep much better, and the strain in my muscles has vanished. I'm 65 years old, my loose teeth are much tighter and I feel like I'm walking around with a younger person's body."

Lee is so convinced of the effectiveness of this simple therapy he states, "Anyone who won't research this method and try it for a month to understand that it works is truly dumber than a rock."

Is a month enough time to reverse chronic conditions that may have existed for several years? In Tara's and Lee's cases it was. Others agree that just one or two months is enough time to bring significant results.

"I thought I was too young for arthritis," says Catalina, of Puerto Vallarta, Mexico, in a posting to www.earthclinic.com, "but my shoulders, hips, knees, feet, and neck were getting achy in the joints. After two months of oil pulling, all aches are gone, and have not returned six months later. Also my keratosis pilaris (a chronic skin disease) has cleared up, my skin is softer, and my facial wrinkles have markedly decreased. My teeth are whiter, my tongue cleaner and pinker, my gums are pink, the dark circles under my eyes have lessened, and I have less gray hair. Yes, it's true! Both my husband and I have noticed a 50 percent decrease in gray hair, with brown hair returning."

Like Lee, Catalina is also feeling younger. "I'm sleeping more soundly, have more energy, and generally feel better all around. I know this all sounds too good to be true, but after nine months of oil pulling, I don't see how this can be attributed to a placebo effect. Something is working. I will never stop oil pulling." Catalina agrees with Lee, "Give it 30 days and you will see results."

As Tara stated, and Lee and Catalina would probably agree, "Oil pulling gave me my life back!"

WHAT'S IT ALL ABOUT?

The changes described by Tara, Lee, and Catalina seem incredible. Could it be possible? Having a background in medicine, I was skeptical. When I first heard about oil pulling, like many, I thought it too simplistic to be of any value. After all, how could rinsing your mouth with oil cure arthritis or chronic fatigue? It just didn't make sense. What compounded the mystery was that most people who were oil pulling at the time were using sunflower oil. Sunflower oil isn't known to have any special healing properties, so I was ready to dismiss it without further investigation.

Over the following months, however, I kept running across this "oil pulling," and many people seemed convinced that there was something to it. Testimonies sounded sincere and convincing. These were first-hand accounts, not stories told to them by their sister's best friend's brother. By nature and by training, I'm very skeptical of so-called "miracle cures," and question every unproven health treatment—especially those in the natural health field. I have seen many "natural" treatments that turned out to be totally worthless. Usually they were promoted by some business as a means to lighten other people's pockets and fill their own. To me, this seemed like just another one of these phony cures. However, I began hearing so much about it that I decided to look closer and see what all the fuss was about.

I did a search on the Internet and found several websites describing the technique, along with many testimonies like those described earlier. I looked for some technical information, but couldn't find a thing. But one thing that impressed me was that none of these websites were selling anything related to oil pulling. They were not promoting it for profit, but simply to educate. Most new therapies and products have some commercial connection. It was nice to see that this was not the case.

Oil pulling, as I learned, was not a new invention or some clever marketing gimmick. It was a technique practiced in Ayurvedic medicine and had been used for generations. In recent years it has gained attention due to the work of Dr. F. Karach, M.D. Dr. Karach had refined the technique and incorporated it in his practice with remarkable results. He presented a lecture in the Ukraine describing his technique, which stirred up interest, especially in India where Ayurvedic medicine holds a position of great respect.

As I started reading the material, I soon realized that there was a very logical, science-based reason for the incredible healing effects associated with oil pulling, but no one else seemed to know what it was. I read all types of explanations as to why oil pulling works—it sucks toxins out of the bloodstream through a vein under the tongue, the mouth absorbs essential fatty acids from the oil, it activates special detoxifying enzymes in the saliva, it balances the body's charkras or chi energy flow, and so forth—all of which have little credibility. People didn't know why or how it worked, so to the best of their understanding they created explanations. I was surprised that no one ever mentioned what, to me, seemed to be the most obvious explanation.

YOUR MOUTH IS A WINDOW TO YOUR BODY

Some years earlier I wrote a book on the health benefits of coconut oil, titled *The Coconut Oil Miracle*. While doing research for that book I discovered the key to unlocking the mystery behind oil pulling. There was a great deal of research in medical and dental journals describing the link between oral health and systemic disease. I began an in-depth search uncovering hundreds of studies, and the more I searched, the more evidence I found to validate the effectiveness of oil pulling as a therapeutic tool.

Just as the eyes are viewed as the window to the soul, the mouth is a window to the body. By looking into the mouth, you can tell a great deal about a person's health. Cavity-riddled teeth, swollen and inflamed gums, bad breath, discoloration on the tongue, receding and bleeding gums, yellowed teeth, plaque and tarter buildup, dental fillings, missing teeth, etc., are all signs reflecting a person's state of health. The mouth is part of the digestive tract. When you look inside the mouth, you are seeing a representation of the condition of the entire intestinal tract. If the mouth is healthy, the intestines will be healthy. If your teeth and gums are deteriorating, then you are deteriorating. Our mouths can reveal evidence for diabetes, measles, leukemia, syphilis, AIDS, bulimia, irritable bowel syndrome, heartburn, cancer, and other maladies.[1]

The bacteria and other microorganisms that inhabit our mouths influence our health and are influenced by our health. Disease influences the type of bacteria that grow on the lining of the mouth, tongue, and throat. Early stages of cancer, for instance, can be detected by the types of bacteria present. Some mouths contain more harmful organisms than others. If these organisms find a way into the bloodstream, they can wreak havoc on the entire body.

I knew that bacteria from oral infections could enter the bloodstream and cause infections in other parts of the body. There are a number of studies that document this. What I wanted to learn is how bacteria in the mouth could cause or trigger arthritis, chronic fatigue, diabetes, and all the other health conditions for which people claim oil pulling is useful.

Oil pulling is apparently an excellent method for improving oral health. It soaks up or "pulls" disease-causing bacteria and their toxins out from around the teeth and gums, cleaning the mouth far better than any toothbrush or mouthwash. There are countless testimonies on the effectiveness of oil pulling in whitening teeth, removing plaque, relieving inflammation and infection from gums, and improving the overall health of the mouth. If the mouth is a window to one's health, then oil pulling could conceivably have an effect on the health of the entire body.

Another clue to the legitimacy of oil pulling comes from Dr. Joseph Phillips, D.D.S., a periodontist from Ossco, Wisconsin. Over 60 years ago, Dr. Phillips developed a technique for "pulling" infections and germs from the mouth using a method very different from oil pulling, but with remarkably similar results. His method is known as the *Phillips Blotting Technique,* and is still practiced today. This technique is reported to eliminate bad breath, cavities, plaque, tartar, and gum disease. It pulls harmful bacteria and toxins that cause oral infections out of the mouth. These infections, if not treated properly, could spread to other parts of the body, causing any number of infectious and chronic diseases. The Phillips Blotting Technique is reported to not only improve dental health but also systemic problems like arthritis and dermatitis.

In the Phillips Blotting Technique a specially designed toothbrush is used. The blotting brush looks like a traditional toothbrush, but the bristles are textured and more densely grouped, and it is held differently.

Teeth are not brushed, but blotted, like a painter's brush. By capillary action, plaque-forming bacteria are drawn away from the teeth and gums and into the bristles.

Those who have used the Phillips Blotting Technique have reported complete recovery from gum disease and tooth decay. The Phillips Blotting Technique was designed specifically to improve oral health, which apparently it does very well, but as a consequence of removing disease-causing bacteria from the mouth, various other health problems also improve.

I was amazed at the similarity between oil pulling and the Phillips Blotting Technique. Both are very effective in removing troublesome bacteria from the mouth and improving dental health. People have reported remarkable recoveries from dental and systemic health problems from both techniques. Oil pulling, however, has several advantages: you don't have to purchase and use special blotting toothbrushes, you can oil pull just about any time and anywhere, and it is much more thorough. A brush cannot reach the surface of every crook and cranny in the mouth. Oil swished in the mouth, however, comes into contact with 100 percent of the surfaces of your teeth, gums, and other soft tissues, thus the cleansing effect is more thorough.

A SIMPLE CURE

Unlike most forms of medical treatment, oil pulling is very simple, completely harmless, and inexpensive. The cost is the price of a daily spoonful of vegetable oil—cheaper than even a vitamin tablet. Yet it is one of the most powerful forms of therapy I have ever encountered. As a nutritionist and naturopathic physician, I've become familiar with many forms of therapy. After studying and using oil pulling myself, I can say that it beats just about any other form of natural therapy hands down.

One of the things that really impressed me during my research was the multitude of testimonies on the effectiveness of oil pulling. This is important. While a few positive responses could be chalked up to wishful thinking or the placebo effect, there were just too many on oil pulling to ignore. The sheer volume of positive results demonstrates that there is something happening; it isn't all due to mass hysteria or mind over matter.

The most obvious result of oil pulling is improved dental health. Teeth become whiter, gums pinker and healthier looking, and breath fresher. That alone makes it worthwhile. What is really remarkable is that the health benefits don't stop there. Many health problems, including those which medical science has yet to find cures for, are also improved or completely cured. Oil pulling has the potential to help with just about any illness or chronic condition.

Below is a list of some of the most common conditions people have reported that respond to oil pulling:

Acne	Diabetes
Allergies	Eczema
Arthritis	Hemorrhoids
Asthma	Hypertension
Back and Neck Pain	Insomnia
Bad Breath	Migraine Headaches
Bronchitis	Mucous Congestion
Chronic Fatigue	Peptic Ulcers
Colitis	PMS
Crohn's Disease	Periodontal Disease
Constipation	Bleeding Gums
Dental Cavities	Sinusitis
Dermatitis	Tooth Abscess

In addition to the above-mentioned conditions, medical studies have indicated that the following can also be directly related to oral health and may respond to oil pulling therapy:

Acidosis	Gallbladder Disease
Adult Respiratory Distress	Gout
Syndrome (ARDS)	Heart Disease
Atherosclerosis	Hyperglycemia
Blood Disorders	Infertility
Brain Abscess	Kidney Disease
Cancer	Liver Disease
Emphysema	Meningitis

Nerve Disorders	Preterm/Low Birth Weight Babies
Osteoporosis	Psychotic Episodes
Paget's Disease	Stroke
Pneumonia	Toxic Shock Syndrome
Preeclampsia	Many types of Infectious Disease

Basically all areas of the body can be affected by the health of our mouths and the types of organisms that live there.

THE NEW OIL PULLING THERAPY

During my research, I was impressed with the multitude of scientific research that tied into oil pulling. Although there were few studies on the effects of oil pulling itself, there were hundreds of studies linking dental health to systemic and chronic disease. There was a sound scientific basis for the many positive effects observed from oil pulling.

I began oil pulling myself, using coconut oil. To get quick results, I started by pulling three times a day, on an empty stomach, once before each meal. The results were almost immediate, but unlike anything I ever expected. My sinuses began draining heavily and my throat became hoarse, which eventually progressed to laryngitis. At first, I thought I had come down with the flu, but I hadn't had a cold or the flu for more than 8 years, and no one in my family or my workplace were sick. What was odd about this "flu" was that I didn't feel sick. My energy level was normal, I slept fine, and didn't have any of the usual aches and pains associated with the flu. I soon realized that it wasn't the flu, but a cleansing reaction due to the oil pulling. I had read about others who experienced healing crises when they started. What really convinced me was when I came across the experience of a man who developed the exact same symptoms as I was having. After a few days the symptoms left. New symptoms would surface from time to time. I developed a toothache that lasted for one day and as quickly as it appeared, it vanished. A couple of days later, another tooth began to ache and that, too, was gone a day later. Occasionally I would have a coughing fit and expel chunks of mucous. My body was cleansing, ridding itself of garbage.

I found this very interesting, because I have gone through many "detox" programs, and oil pulling was working as well as the best of them in purging junk from my system, and, I must say, it was doing this with far less effort. Oil pulling, for instance, is far easier than going on a water fast for three weeks. My mouth was definitely cleaner and healthier looking. My teeth became slightly whiter, my tongue displayed a healthy pink color, and my breath was clean and fresh.

The most noticeable change was evidenced on my face. For the past 30 years I have struggled with a chronic case of dermatitis. It first became evident when I was in college. My face and chest would flare up periodically, becoming a bright red. Skin would peel and flake off, and become very itchy and even painful. Sometimes the inflammation became so severe the skin would crack and ooze. I went to several dermatologists but none of them knew what it was, and didn't show much concern, telling me simply to use cortisone creams to reduce the swelling and live with it.

As the years passed, the condition grew more severe and more frequent. It got to the point that my face and chest were inflamed nearly 24 hours a day with some days that were more severe than others. I tried every cream, lotion, medicine, dietary supplement, and herb I could find, without results. I even tested for allergies and food sensitivities, but still no luck.

I started to take better care of my health and learned about diet, nutrition, and natural health. My diet completely changed. This took several years, but as my diet improved so did my skin condition. Inflammation subsided and flare-ups became less frequent. The improvement was substantial, but not complete. I went through several detox programs, including many water and juice fasts lasting up to 30 days, but they didn't solve the problem. Slight redness and flaky skin persisted.

I noticed that when my immune system was depressed due to excessive stress, infection, or consuming too much sugar, the rash would flare up again. Certain chemicals, particularly MSG, would also depress my immune system, causing a flare-up. Whenever I went out to eat I could tell if the restaurant used MSG, because within a couple of hours my face would break out in a horrible, itchy rash that would last for several days.

From the very first day I started oil pulling, the redness in my face completely vanished, and I've had no flare-ups since, even when I splurged (at Christmas) and ate much more sugar than I usually do. This was remarkable! Oil pulling has done more for this problem than any of the other detox methods I have ever tried, including the extended fasts. I now believe that the rash was caused by bacteria imbedded in my mouth. When my immune system was challenged, the bacteria were allowed to proliferate. It was probably the toxins released by the bacteria that caused my skin to react and break out. At that point, I knew oil pulling worked and was potentially the most powerful method anyone can use to improve his or her health naturally.

Another remarkable thing happened. All my life I have suffered from severe dandruff. It wasn't just a few flakes here and there, it was massive excess skin coming off in huge flakes. Nothing I tried could stop it. All I could do was keep it under control with medicated shampoo. Ordinary shampoos and soaps didn't do a thing. I needed special shampoos with anti-dandruff medication. Once I discovered the benefits of coconut oil, I was able to replace the medicated shampoo with coconut oil. I would massage the oil into my scalp, let it soak in for several minutes, and then wash it out using ordinary soap. I had to use either medicated shampoo or coconut oil regularly to avoid a pending snowstorm. If I stopped using coconut oil (or medicated shampoo) for more than a week, the dandruff came roaring back with a vengeance.

Since oil pulling had worked so well on my face, I thought maybe it would have an affect on my chronic dandruff as well. So as an experiment, I stopped using coconut oil and washed my hair with an ordinary bar of soap. Normally dandruff would start to return after about a week. One week went by, and there was no sign of dandruff. After two weeks, still no sign of dandruff. I was amazed! After three weeks, my scalp was still 95 percent dandruff-free. I have never, without the aid of coconut oil or medicated shampoo, been able to go this long without experiencing severe dandruff—ever! Dandruff is caused by a fungus (*Malassezia globosa*) which grows in the skin and affects up to 90 percent of the population to one degree or another. Various factors such as immune function and diet can influence the rate of dandruff. Anti-fungal medicated shampoos can normally keep dandruff under control. And, apparently, so can oil pulling!

Something else happened. A wart that I've had on my face for at least two decades suddenly disappeared. Warts are caused by a virus (*human papillomavirus*). Apparently, oil pulling is like a vacuum cleaner that sucks viruses, bacteria, and fungus out of the body. Some health care practitioners believe that most all illnesses are caused by infections. If this is true, then oil pulling is potentially one of the most powerful natural healing tools available.

I continued researching, experimenting, and telling others about it. Over time I took the oil pulling method taught by Dr. Karach (mentioned earlier in this chapter) and combined it with what I learned about the science behind it. I refined it, improved it, and created a more complete method of detoxification, which I call "Dr. Fife's Oil Pulling Therapy." This book isn't just about oil pulling, it is a complete course in oil pulling therapy.

Chapter 2

Bacteria, Fungus, and Tooth Decay

WHAT'S LIVING IN YOUR MOUTH?

Your mouth is like a tropical rain forest. It is hot, humid, and maintains a fairly constant temperature year round. Like a rain forest, it is teaming with life—bacteria, viruses, fungi, and protozoa. Although you can't see them, your mouth is home to billions of microorganisms. By far the greatest number of organisms that populate your mouth are bacteria: short ones, fat ones, long ones, skinny ones—they're all represented. You have so many bacteria living in your mouth that their population far exceeds the number of people living on the earth.

Food for these little buggers is plentiful. What do they like to eat? They like to eat pizza, ice cream, and donuts! What you eat, they eat. They thrive on a diet of sugar and other carbohydrates—their preferred foods. They love the little tasty morsels that get caught between your teeth or become wedged in the folds between your cheek and gums, where they can nibble on them happily for hours. It is no wonder that in such an ideal environment, our mouths are home to so many creatures.

Your mouth, in essence, is a mini-ecosystem. The weather forecast is the same every day: 95° F (35° C) unless we are ill, with 100 percent humidity. Microorganisms are selective. They don't colonize your mouth in a random way; they form communities. Like an ecosystem in a tropical forest where some creatures prefer to live on the ground, others in the trees, or on water, the microorganisms in our mouths also select their own living space. Some prefer life on the teeth, others prefer the space between the gums and teeth, others prefer the roof of the mouth, and yet others prefer the pockets in the front or on the back of the tongue. Although they may touch each other, each micro-community contains a distinct population.

Each person has a set of unique communities of microorganisms living in their mouths. A person living in London has different micro-communities from someone living in New York, who in turn, has different groups of organisms than people living in New Orleans. Even among family members, communities differ. Despite close contact, a husband and wife have their own distinct microbial populations.

The micro-communities in our mouths are unique for each individual because the environment or ecology of everyone's mouth is unique. Our oral environment is a product of our diet, lifestyle, genetics, gender, etc. Stress, for example, can impact our immune system, which in turn affects the microbes in our mouths. Hormone levels also have an influence; certain hormones encourage the growth of specific organisms. People who are subclinically dehydrated most of the time have decreased saliva production; saliva contains buffers and enzymes that profoundly affect the environment and the microbe population. Smoking and alcohol consumption also have an impact. One of the biggest factors is diet. Sugar and other carbohydrates act like fertilizer in your garden; bacteria and yeasts proliferate in their presence.

Our health also affects the types of organisms that inhabit our mouths. High blood sugar, as seen in diabetics, encourages the growth of certain mouth-dwelling bacteria. Overweight individuals have different microbes in their mouths than normal-weight people. Medical researchers are even able to identify certain health conditions based on the micro-communities in the mouth. So you can see there are many factors that influence the micro-populations in our mouths.

Microorganisms begin to inhabit the mouth as soon as we are born. While the mouth and digestive tract of newborns is sterile, they are quickly colonized by microflora in the air, from contact with parents and siblings, and from things they randomly stick in their mouths.

People have an incredibly large amount of bacteria growing in their mouths. In fact, humans have more bacteria in their mouths than dogs do. Considering all the disgusting places where dogs like to stick their muzzles, their mouths are amazingly clean. You would pick up

Inside Your Mouth

Cells lining the inside of our mouths replace themselves every three to seven days.

Bacteria in the human mouth fall into two categories (a) planktonic or free-floating, which can be found in the saliva, and (b) biofilm, the bacteria that colonize on the surfaces of the mouth, such as teeth and tongue.

The human mouth harbors over 600 types of bacteria. The amount of total bacteria is estimated to be around 10 billion.

Anaerobic bacteria produce enzymes and toxins as by-products, which damage and irritate the gums, causing inflammation and bleeding.

Brushing only reaches 60 percent of the surfaces of your teeth, leaving plaque in hard-to-reach areas such as in-between teeth.

more germs from kissing your spouse on the lips than you would from kissing the mouth of a drooling dog! Disgusting for sure, but true. Dogs have antibodies in their saliva that are not found in the human mouth. These antibodies kill disease-causing germs.

"I used to do a laboratory exercise in my classroom," says Roberta M. Meehan, Ph.D., "Every semester in microbiology, the students aseptically swabbed a newborn's mouth and a dog's mouth." You would expect a newborn baby to have minimal bacteria in its mouth, especially compared to a dog. "Everyone was in awe. The baby's mouth was full of bacteria, but the dog's mouth was relatively bacteria-free. And it worked every semester—any veterinarian will validate this."

It is hard to imagine the huge number of bacteria that live in our mouths. A tiny piece of dental plaque small enough to fit on the end of a toothpick holds between ten million to 100 million bacteria. Our bodies are teaming with microscopic life. No matter how hard we may try to get rid of them, there are more bacteria in and on us than there are cells in our bodies. The intestine alone is home to about 100 trillion bacteria, which outnumber all the cells in the human body ten to one. Many of the same bacteria that live in our mouths also take up residence in our intestines and on our skin. Many others, however, are found nowhere else, preferring the warm, moist climate of the oral cavity. There are over 600 different species of bacteria living in our mouths, along with hundreds of species of viruses, fungi, and protozoa. New species are continually being discovered. Only a fraction of them have been studied in any detail. The rest we know little about, and even less how they might affect our dental or overall health.

SALIVA

Some oral bacteria are relatively benign, and in some cases even helpful. Others are more aggressive and troublesome, causing cavities and gum disease. One of the most troublesome critters is *Streptococcus mutans* (S. mutans). It is the primary cause of the cavities in our teeth. This species, and others like it, thrive on sugar and refined carbohydrates. As part of the bacteria's digestive process, sugar is converted into acid and released as a waste product. This acid erodes the enamel of the teeth, weakening the protective covering on the teeth and initiating decay. This is why people who eat a lot of sweets have a lot of cavities.

No matter how often you brush your teeth, floss, and attempt to sterilize your mouth with oral disinfectants, the effect you have on the microbial population is only minor. Most organisms survive the treatment and quickly multiply and repopulate this ideal habitat. The battle against these squatters is constant.

If it wasn't for your saliva, your teeth would rot and your mouth would be covered with infections regardless of what you did. Saliva is essential for the digestion of food as well as keeping our mouths healthy. It contains a complex mixture of enzymes, buffers, antibodies, and nutrients that fight off disease and keep the teeth and gums in good working order.

19

Bacteria Commonly Found

Bacterium	Skin	Conjunctiva	Nose
Staphylococcus epidermidis	++	+	++
Staphylococcus aureus*	+	+/-	+
Streptococcus mitis	-	-	-
Streptococcus salivarius	-	-	-
Streptococcus mutans*	-	-	-
Enterococcus faecalis*	-	-	-
Streptococcus pneumoniae*	-	+/-	+/-
Streptococcus pyogenes*	+/-	+/-	-
Neisseria sp.	-	+	+
Neisseria meningitides*	-	-	+
Veillonellae sp.	-	-	-
Enterobacteriaceae* (Escherichia coli)	-	+/-	+/-
Proteus sp.	-	+/-	+
Pseudomonas aeruginosa*	-	-	-
Haemophilus influenzae*	-	+/-	+
Bacteroides sp.*	-	-	-
Bifidobacterium bifidum	-	-	-
Lactobacillus sp.	-	-	-
Clostridium sp.*	-	-	-
Clostridium tetani	-	-	-
Corynebacteria	++	+	++
Mycobacteria	+	-	+/-
Actinomycetes	-	-	-
Spirochetes	-	-	-
Mycoplasmas	-	-	-

Key: ++ = nearly 100 percent   + = common   +/- = rare   - = none
* = potential pathogen (in situ)

The skin and mucous membranes of the human body are in constant contact with the environment and become readily colonized by certain microbial species. The combination and number of organisms regularly found at any location is exceedingly complex. Bacteria are the most numerous. The distribution of the bacteria is shown in the table above. This table lists only a fraction of the total bacterial species that occur as normal flora of humans and does not express the total number or concentration of bacteria at any site.

On the Human Body

Pharynx	Mouth	Lower Intestine	Anterior Urethra	Vagina
++	++	+	++	++
+	+	++	+/-	+
+	++	+/-	+	+
++	++	-	-	-
+	++	-	-	-
+/-	+	++	+	+
+	+	-	-	+/-
+	+	+/-	-	+/-
++	+	-	+	+
++	+	-	-	+
-	+	+/-	-	-
+/-	+	++	+	+
+	+	+	+	+
+/-	+/-	+	+/-	-
+	+	-	-	-
-	-	++	+	+/-
-	-	++	-	-
-	+	++	-	++
-	+/-	++	-	-
-	-	+/-	-	-
+	+	+	+	+
+/-	-	+	+	-
+	+	+	+/-	+
+	++	++	-	-
+	+	+	+/-	+

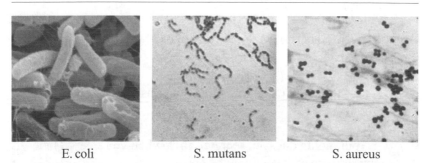

E. coli   S. mutans   S. aureus

Source: Todar, K. *Todar's Online Textbook of Bacteriology*, University of Wisconsin-Madison Department of Bacteriology.

21

Enzymes in the mouth begin the process of digesting the foods we eat. Carbohydrates, the primary nutritional component of grains, fruits, and vegetables, are broken down into smaller units and simple sugars by salivary enzymes. Bacteria in the mouth feed on these same carbohydrates and sugars, producing potentially harmful acids. Saliva dilutes the acids and neutralizes them with chemical buffers. This way, a more neutral pH is maintained.

Saliva contains unique antibodies and antimicrobial compounds that help control the growth of certain pathogenic organisms. Unfortunately, these compounds don't kill all troublemakers, and the mouth and the saliva still harbor many potentially harmful germs.

Saliva also contains a high concentration of certain mineral ions, particularly calcium and phosphate, the main ingredients of teeth. Microscopic lesions in tooth enamel can be remineralized, and thus repaired, by saliva.

Saliva is produced throughout the day. At certain times, such as when a meal is being eaten, saliva excretion increases. At night, when you sleep, virtually no saliva is produced. People who do not drink enough liquids during the day become chronically dehydrated. As a result, they do not produce enough saliva to adequately protect their teeth from decay. People who are chronically dehydrated or have medical conditions that reduce saliva output have a significantly greater amount of tooth decay and gum disease.

Saliva

We produce approximately 1 liter (34 ounces) of saliva a day.

One teaspoon (5 ml) of saliva contains about 2.5 billion bacterial cells.

Your mouth does not secrete saliva when you sleep. This is why sleeping with your mouth open will result in a dry mouth.

The pH Scale

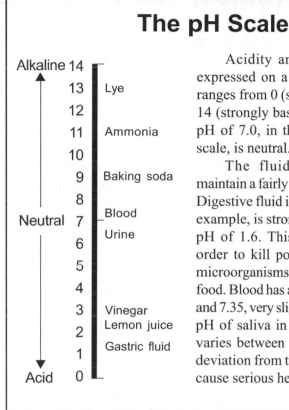

Alkaline 14

13   Lye

12

11   Ammonia

10

9   Baking soda

8

Neutral 7   Blood

6   Urine

5

4

3   Vinegar

2   Lemon juice

1   Gastric fluid

Acid 0

Acidity and alkalinity are expressed on a pH scale, which ranges from 0 (strongly acidic) to 14 (strongly basic or alkaline). A pH of 7.0, in the middle of this scale, is neutral.

The fluids in our body maintain a fairly constant pH level. Digestive fluid in the stomach, for example, is strongly acidic with a pH of 1.6. This is necessary in order to kill potentially harmful microorganisms and to help digest food. Blood has a pH between 7.45 and 7.35, very slightly alkaline. The pH of saliva in a healthy person varies between 6.0 and 7.4. Any deviation from these readings can cause serious health problems.

Another problem is the over-consumption of sugar and refined carbohydrates. Sugar encourages the growth of acid-producing bacteria. Bicarbonate ions in our saliva possess the ability to counteract the acid produced in most traditional or ancestral diets. Consequently, our ancestors had far fewer cavities than we do. Most diets today contain way too much processed sugar and refined carbohydrates, which are easily transformed into sugar by digestive enzymes in our saliva. The acid produced from eating a high-carb diet, increases beyond the natural ability of saliva to control. Acid-producing bacteria like *Streptococcus mutans* tend to overpopulate the mouths of those who eat high-carb diets.

COMMON ORAL PROBLEMS
Halitosis

Are you troubled with chronic bad breath? If so, you can put the blame on the bacteria residing in your mouth. Certain bacteria that can dominate the back portion of the top of your tongue can produce halitosis—otherwise known as bad breath.

About 20 percent of the population suffers from halitosis. Halitosis differs from the temporary mouth odors caused by foods. It is usually chronic, being the product of the type of bacteria inhabiting the mouth. Although not really a dental condition, halitosis does reflect the health and environment of the mouth. A healthy mouth, in a healthy body, should have no offensive odor.

The bacteria that colonize the back portion of the top of your tongue vary from person to person. Halitosis is caused by certain species of bacteria that are not found to any extent in those people with fresh breath.

Halitosis in itself is not considered a serious condition, but it is annoying and can interfere with social life. Foul breath can also be a sign of tooth decay or gum disease.

Dentists recommend that we not only brush our teeth, but also our gums and our tongue to scrape off the offending bacteria. Antiseptic mouthwashes are also recommended, but these measures are only temporary since the bacteria quickly reestablish themselves.

Oral Bacteria

There are more bacteria in your mouth than there are people on the Earth.

The average toilet seat harbors fewer bacteria per square inch than the human mouth!

There are more bacteria in your mouth right now than there are on the bottom of the average shoe.

A Healthy Tooth

The surfaces of the teeth are covered by a very hard, dense material called enamel. This is the hardest tissue in the human body. Below the gums, the tooth roots are not covered with enamel, but a thin, hard layer called the cementum.

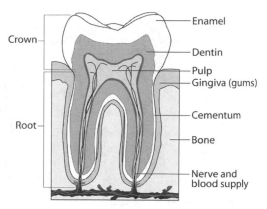

Underneath the enamel and cementum lies the dentin. Dentin is less hard than enamel and cementum, and similar in composition to bone. It makes up the majority of the tooth. The terms "dentist" and "dentistry" are derived from the word dentin. At the center of the tooth is the pulp, which contains the nerve and blood vessels.

Dental Caries (Cavities)

Dental caries, or cavities as they are commonly called, are the result of tooth decay. If left untreated, cavities continue to grow, causing pain and ultimately death of the tooth. Tooth decay is one of the most common chronic diseases in the world. An estimated 90 percent of schoolchildren worldwide have experienced some level of tooth decay.

Tooth decay is initiated by acid-producing bacteria that feed on sugars (sucrose, fructose, and glucose). Carbohydrates, which are broken down into sugars by digestive enzymes in the saliva, and sugary foods feed these bacteria. Consequently, acid levels in the mouth increase.

Most cavities begin in the hard enamel surrounding the exposed portions of our teeth and gradually work their way down into the underlying softer dentin. The enamel is the most vulnerable to cavities simply because it is in close contact with bacteria and mineral-dissolving acids. Our teeth prefer a slightly alkaline environment and are very sensitive to changes in pH. Teeth are an extension of our skeletons,

Progression of Tooth Decay

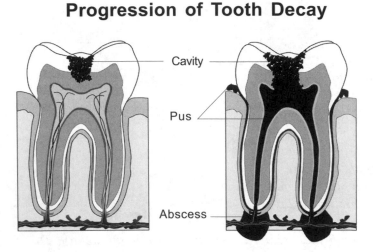

Cavity

Pus

Abscess

Cavities eat their way through the enamel and into the dentin and pulp. Once bacteria enter the pulp, an abscess can develop.

and like bones, are living tissue that are continually being remineralized and demineralized. In a very low acid or slightly alkaline environment, remineralization proceeds faster than demineralization and the teeth become denser and stronger. When the pH at the surface of the teeth drops below 5.5 (mildly acidic), demineralization of the enamel becomes faster than remineralization, resulting in a net loss of mineral density. As the enamel becomes demineralized, bacteria are able to penetrate into the teeth causing decay.

When the gums are healthy, cavities in the root are less likely to develop because the surfaces are not accessible to acid-producing bacteria. Cementum, which is the thin hard layer that covers the tooth root, is exposed when gums pull away from the teeth. Exposed cementum is more vulnerable to demineralization than enamel. It begins to demineralize at a pH of only 6.7. When gums recede, roots are left vulnerable to decay.

If a cavity has only penetrated the enamel, there may be no pain. If the cavity extends into the dentin, the tooth may become sensitive to hot, cold, or sweet foods. When the pulp is involved, pain can be continuous and throbbing. If left untreated, an abscess can develop and the tooth will die. At this stage the dentist will either perform a root canal or extract the tooth.

Dental Plaque

Plaque is the accumulation of mucous, food particles, bacteria and other microorganisms, and their products, which form a sticky, cream or yellow-colored mass on tooth surfaces. Unlike tarter, dental plaque is soft and easily removed by brushing and flossing the teeth. The accumulation of plaque can lead to periodontal disease (gum disease), as well as tooth decay.

Plaque begins to form on the teeth within 20 minutes after eating. It tends to accumulate in areas that are not easily accessible to brushing, such as between and behind teeth.

Calculus (Tartar)

Calculus or tartar is a mineral deposit that develops on teeth. It is basically plaque that, over time, becomes mineralized. Calculus is hard and firmly attached to the tooth. It cannot be removed by brushing or flossing. It usually requires special dental tools for removal.

Calculus can form above or below the gum line. The bacteria that form plaque and stick to calculus can irritate and inflame the gums, leading to gum or periodontal disease.

Gingivitis

Gingiva is the medical term used for our gums. Gingivitis is inflammation of the gums. It is the first stage of gum disease (periodontal disease). Common features of gingivitis are red and swollen gums and the presence of bleeding while brushing and flossing. Gingivitis develops as bacteria and toxins in plaque irritate the gums.

Gingivitis is widespread. Worldwide, by the time children reach adolescence, 70-90 percent are affected. Gingivitis is usually painless and not necessarily recognizable to the untrained eye, consequently, most people don't realize they have it. If left untreated it can develop into periodontitis.

Periodontal Disease

Common features of peri-odontal disease are in-flamed and receding gums, presence of plaque, and bleeding while brush-ing. Chronic inflamma-tion can cause degenera-tion of the bone.

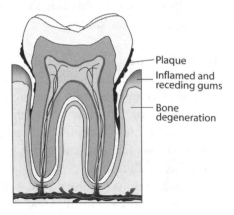

Plaque

Inflamed and receding gums

Bone degeneration

Periodontitis

Periodontitis, also known as pyorrhea, results from chronic gingivitis. It is a more advanced stage of gum disease. Bacteria, and the toxins they produce, cause the gums to become infected, swollen and tender. The infected gums pull away from the teeth and form pockets. Bacteria and plaque spread and grow below the gum line. Toxins from bacteria and the body's enzymes fighting the infection start to break down the bone and connective tissue that hold teeth in place. If not treated, the bones, gums, and connective tissue that support the teeth are destroyed. The teeth may eventually become loose and have to be removed.

Signs of periodontal disease include red or swollen gums, tender or bleeding gums, receding gum line, loose teeth, pain while chewing, sensitive teeth, and bad breath that won't go away. Tooth decay usually accompanies periodontal disease. In the US, and likely in Canada and the UK as well, periodontitis affects about 50 percent of adults over 30 years of age.

Dental Abscess

An abscess is a localized collection of pus in a cavity formed by the disintegration of tissue. Abscesses are usually caused by microorganisms that invade the tissues. A tooth abscess typically originates from dead pulp tissue, usually caused by untreated tooth decay, cracked teeth, or extensive periodontal disease. A failed root canal treatment may also create an abscess.

Abscesses can be acute or chronic. The difference depends on how rapidly they form and how effective the body is in defending itself. An acute abscess is characterized by pain, swelling, and fever. A chronic abscess may be painless. In fact, a person may be unaware of its presence even as it continues to grow inside the jawbone.

Failure to treat an abscess can lead to serious infection, which can spread into surrounding tissue and penetrate to the bone marrow of the jaw. A serious infection can dump large quantities of bacteria into the bloodstream, causing septicemia (blood poisoning).

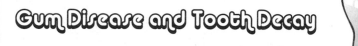

Gum Disease and Tooth Decay

Five percent of babies have some tooth decay by 9 months of age, 15 percent by 12 months, and 17 percent by 4 years of age.

Moderate periodontal disease is found in 40 percent of children over 12 years of age.

Oral conditions, such as gingivitis and chronic periodontitis, are found worldwide and are among the most prevalent microbial diseases of mankind. According to a study in the British medical journal *The Lancet*, periodontal disease affects up to 90 percent of the population worldwide.[1]

According to the U.S. Centers for Disease Control and Prevention (CDC), nine out of every 10 people have tooth decay. One in 20 middle-aged adults and one in three adults over the age of 65 have lost all of their natural teeth.

Periodontal Disease Assessment

Do you have periodontal disease? Many people are unaware that they have gum disease. The absence of pain, obvious inflammation, or tooth decay is no guarantee you are free from periodontal disease. To test your risk, answer each of the following questions as truthfully as possible. Keep track of your total points (shown in brackets) and evaluate your score at the end of the test.

How old are you?   <40 [5]   40-65[10]   >65[15]
Do you use tobacco?   No[5]   Yes[15]
Have you seen a dentist in the past two years?   No[10]   Yes[5]
How often do you floss?   Daily [5]   Weekly [10]   Seldom [15]
Do you have any of the following health conditions?
(Heart disease, osteoporosis, osteopenia, high stress, or diabetes)
                                                                            No[5]   Yes[25]
Do you have chronic bad breath or a persistent metallic taste in your mouth?   No[5]   Yes[15]
How many dental fillings do you have?
                                        None[5]   1-3 [10]   4 or more[15]
Do your gums bleed after brushing?   No[5]   Yes[55]
Do you have any loose teeth?   No[5]   Yes[55]
Do you have receding gums or do your teeth look longer?
                                                                No[5]   Yes[55]
Have you had any adult teeth extracted?   No[5]   Yes[55]
Do you have any root canalled teeth?   No[5]   Yes[55]

Your Periodontal Disease Risk Score

Low Risk: 75 or less points
Medium Risk: 80 to105 points
High Risk: 110 or more points

If you scored 75 points or less, your risk of having periodontal disease is low. At 80-105 points you have medium risk, or likely, mild periodontal disease. If you scored 110 or more points, your risk of having periodontal disease is high, and the higher your score the more severe the condition is likely to be.

Even if you have a high score, your risk can be significantly reduced by proper dental care and regular oil pulling.

Chapter 3

All Disease Starts in the Mouth

It may sound unbelievable, but with few exceptions, all disease starts in the mouth. I'm not talking about conditions caused by genetics or physical or emotional trauma; I'm talking about the majority of illness and disease that plague the human race, including chronic degenerative disease. It is through the mouth that all disease gets its start.

Think about it for a moment. Our mouths and nasal passages are the passageways into our bodies. It is through the mouth and sinuses that we take in air and get nourishment—the two things most vital to our survival and existence. This is also the passageway into our bodies for disease-causing toxins and germs.

Without oxygen, we could only survive for a matter of minutes. The quality of the air that we breathe can affect our health in many ways. Polluted air, toxic gas, tobacco smoke, allergy-causing pollen, and germs can all have an impact on our health.

Likewise, what we put into our mouths can greatly impact our health. The food we eat nourishes our bodies. Inadequate food intake or poor dietary habits can cause malnutrition and nutritional deficiency diseases, and increase our risk for developing degenerative disease. Too much food, whether nutritious or not, can lead to obesity and a whole host of other problems.

Insufficient water intake or excess coffee, alcohol, and soda intake can lead to acute or chronic dehydration. Drugs, natural toxins in foods, environmental toxins, residual pesticides, chemical food additives, rancid oils, and industrial contaminants can all enter our bodies through the mouth. What we eat and drink has a great impact on the ability of our immune system to keep us healthy. Poor dietary habits weaken the immune system, making us vulnerable to a multitude of health problems. When the immune system is depressed, cancer and infectious disease can take hold. When the immune system is strong, even potentially serious infections caused by wounds or insect bites can be overcome.

Our mouths are also the entryway into our bodies for bacteria, viruses, fungi, and parasites. Hundreds of billions of microscopic organisms inhabit our mouths and digestive tracts. Some of these organisms are beneficial and others are not. However, all are potentially harmful. Even the beneficial organisms can become deadly if they find entrance into the bloodstream. Microbes can seep into the bloodstream through open sores and wounds or though inflamed tissue. Our mouths provide them an easy entryway into the bloodstream.

In the blood these organisms can cause untold harm, causing systemic and localized infections, chronic inflammation, and initiating an autoimmune response that can lead to a multitude of health problems ranging from arthritis to heart disease. So, as you can see, almost all disease in our society starts in our mouths. In this chapter, you will see how the health of your mouth can have a direct impact on the health of your entire body.

THE FOCAL INFECTION THEORY OF DISEASE

A wise farmer always examines an animal's mouth before buying it. He knows that the condition of the animal's mouth reflects the health of its entire body. No farmer in his right mind is going to pay top dollar for an animal with missing teeth or swollen gums. Dental problems signal that other health problems are likely present. This is true with humans as well. This fact was recognized centuries ago and was the basis for the focal infection theory used in dentistry. This theory basically states that an oral infection can influence the health of the entire body. Based on this theory, old-time dentists were inclined to pull all diseased teeth in hopes of preventing disease from spreading to other parts of the body.

The connection between dental and whole-body health was recognized at least 2,700 years ago. It is mentioned in ancient Assyrian and Greek medical texts. Hippocrates, the Greek physician who is considered the father of Western medicine, reports curing a patient of arthritis by pulling an infected tooth.[1] Before the twentieth century, the focal theory of infection was considered to be so obvious it was accepted as a fact. Those who worked with animals knew very well that dental health affected overall health. In humans, when infected teeth were pulled, patients often reported recovery from various other health problems.

So how does tooth decay or swollen gums affect other parts of the body? How can an infected tooth cause arthritis or pneumonia, or precipitate a heart attack or stroke? Who of us are at risk?

If you had the misfortune to be bitten by a dog—bitten hard enough to puncture the skin—what would be one of the first things you would do to treat the wound? The first thing you should do is disinfect the wound: wash it with soap and water to kill any germs that might cause an infection. In fact, we are taught to wash any type of wound to remove germs. Germs from the dog's mouth or the environment can cause a serious infection that can spread throughout the body and can cause serious harm.

As you have learned from the previous chapter, the human mouth contains far more germs than a dog's mouth. Therefore, any wound, lesion, puncture, or opening in the mucous membranes of the mouth could allow germs to enter into the bloodstream and cause an infection. Unlike a wound on your arm, that can be washed and bandaged to keep out germs, the mouth is continually bathed in a microbial soup (saliva), filled with bacteria, viruses, fungi, and parasites. It's like wrapping the wound on your arm with a dirty rag that has been soaked in sewage. The likelihood of an infection is high. So, likewise, is the risk of infection from a lesion in the mouth.

People who have serious dental problems, like advanced gum disease or a tooth abscess, are most likely to pass microbial invaders into the bloodstream, but any cut or ulcer in the mouth can do the same. If you have gingivitis, as most people do to one extent or another, simply brushing your teeth each day causes the gums to bleed.[2] This provides germs an entryway into your bloodstream. Flossing as well, can cause bleeding. Even if your teeth are clean and you have no obvious dental problems, you are still at risk. The tissues of the gums are densely packed with blood vessels, and permeability is considerably increased during inflammation. This allows bacteria to seep through inflamed gum tissue and into the bloodstream, whether an open wound is present or not.[3]

Severe periodontitis can cover a surface area of the mouth equivalent to about 9 square inches. This is roughly the size of your forearm. Think about having an open wound the size of your forearm always exposed, 24 hours a day, to a whole variety of dirt and bacteria. We wash and sterilize the tiniest cut on our skin to avoid infection. But in our mouths we have a huge open lesion bathed in disease-causing bacteria. Common sense will tell you something has got to happen. And it does. Bacteria constantly work their way into our bloodstream causing all sorts of havoc.

Once the germs enter the bloodstream they can end up anywhere—your heart, your lungs, your liver—or they may spread throughout your entire body. Just as some bacteria prefer to live on your teeth or your tongue, those that enter the bloodstream often tend to collect or colonize in certain types of tissues. Consequently, mouth bacteria can lead to localized conditions like arthritis (joints) and endocarditis (heart) as well as systemic disease such as diabetes.

In microbiology there is a maxim that states: "Any microorganism outside of its natural environment should be considered a pathogen." In other words, the bacteria that normally reside in your mouth are just fine residing there. However, if they happen to get into your bloodstream, where they don't belong, they could start a serious infection. Any microbe, no matter how benign it is in the mouth or digestive tract, can become a disease-causing monster if it gets into the bloodstream.

Your mouth harbors hundreds of species of bacteria, viruses, fungi, and protozoa. New species are continually being identified. Most of those that have been discovered we know very little about, let alone how they might affect the body if they get into the bloodstream. Therefore, oral microorganisms can potentially cause or contribute to almost any health problem, even conditions that appear to have no connection to infectious organisms.

THE CONTRIBUTIONS OF
DR. WESTON A. PRICE AND OTHERS

In the late nineteenth and early twentieth centuries, several studies were published in medical journals describing and documenting the focal theory of infection.[4-8] In 1923, Weston A. Price, D.D.S., compiled an extensive two-volume set of books containing a total of 1,174 pages, which documented the focal infection theory in detail and contained numerous case studies. The books were titled *Dental Infections, Oral and Systemic, Volume 1* and *Dental Infections and the Degenerative Diseases, Volume II* (see Bibliography). These books were the cumulation of 25 years of research by Dr. Price and his colleagues.

Dr. Weston A. Price was among the most respected dental researchers of his time. He served as the Chairman of the Research Section of the American Dental Association. His research team consisted of 60 of the nation's leading scientists, including such notable scholars as Charles H. Mayo, M.D., President, Clinical Congress of Surgeons of North America and founder of the Mayo Clinic; Victor C. Vaughan, M.D., Dean of the Medical Department at the University of Michigan and President of the American Medical Association; Frank Billings, M.D., head of the Department of Medicine, University of Chicago; and Milton J. Rosenau, M.D., Professor of Preventive Medicine and Hygiene, Harvard Medical School.

By the early 1900s, the practice and science of dentistry had entered the modern era. Dentists, for instance, had been successfully doing fillings and root canals for many years. A root canal is performed when tooth decay is so advanced that the tooth cannot be saved. Instead of pulling it and replacing it with an artificial one, the dead tooth is allowed to remain in place. The soft pulp in the center of the tooth is drilled out, the inside is disinfected, and the cavity is filled with a hard rubber-like material. The tooth is then sealed and capped. It is assumed that this process removes all of the infection.

After observing many patients, Dr. Price had become suspicious that root canal treated teeth always remained infected. One of his patients was a woman who had arthritis so severe that her joints had become swollen and deformed and was unable to walk; she had been confined to a wheelchair for six years. At the time, dentists knew that arthritis and other illnesses often cleared up if bad teeth were extracted.

Although x-ray pictures of her root canal treated tooth showed no evidence or symptoms of an infection, the tooth was extracted.

The tooth was washed and then surgically embedded under the skin of a rabbit. Within two days the rabbit developed the same type of crippling arthritis as Dr. Price's patient. After 10 days the rabbit died from the infection. The patient, now without the infected tooth, made a miraculous recovery and was able to walk without assistance and go back to doing fine needlework, which she enjoyed. Dr. Price encouraged other patients suffering from untreatable chronic health problems to have their root-filled teeth removed.

Continuing with his research, these extracted teeth were then inserted into rabbits. Eventually he was able to obtain cultures of bacteria from inside the teeth and injected the cultured material into rabbits. In almost every instance, the rabbits developed the same or similar diseases as the patients.

If the patients had kidney trouble, the rabbits developed kidney problems; if eye trouble, the rabbits' eyes became affected; heart trouble, rheumatism, stomach ulcers, bladder infections, ovarian diseases, phlebitis, osteomyelitis, whatever the disease, the rabbits promptly become similarly affected. These infections proved so devastating that most animals died within two weeks.

To prove that not all teeth or foreign objects embedded into the animals would result in disease, healthy, sterile teeth and other sterile objects like coins were also tested. When these objects were embedded under a rabbit's skin, no infections occurred. The rabbits remained in good health.

Dr. Price performed hundreds of experiments. There was a patient who had an enormous cyst around an impacted wisdom tooth. This patient had colitis, which resulted in bowel movements every 30 minutes.

"Government statistics speak of the degenerative diseases frequently as old age diseases, and it is pathetic that so many individuals are slowly dying of old age anywhere from thirty years on."

Weston A. Price, D.D.S.

Rabbits inoculated with the contents of the cyst each developed diarrhea, and several developed severe spastic colitis.

It was very common for a rabbit to develop not only the same type of problem as the patient, but also many other conditions as well. For example, a culture made from an extracted tooth was taken from a patient with arthritis, and subsequently four rabbits were inoculated with the bacteria. All four of the rabbits developed acute rheumatism, but, in addition, two of them contracted liver trouble, one gallbladder lesions, one intestinal difficulty, and two developed brain lesions.

Three rabbits were inoculated with an extracted tooth from a patient who had myositis (muscle inflammation), neuritis (inflammation of peripheral nerves), and chronic low back pain. All three of the rabbits developed rheumatism and liver problems, and two of them developed heart lesions, and intestinal and kidney problems; in addition, one each developed disease of the lungs and gallbladder.

Bacteria can be harmful, but the toxins they expel can be just as harmful or even worse. Dr. Price took bacterial cultures from the tooth of a patient who was suffering from severe colitis that caused bowel movements every 15 minutes. Rabbits inoculated with this culture developed diarrhea as well as stomach, gallbladder, and liver problems. The bacteria were then filtered to remove everything but the toxins they produce. When these toxins were injected into the rabbits, 44 percent developed intestinal trouble, 67 percent liver disturbances, and 33 percent heart problems.

Patients suffering from chronic conditions who had their infected teeth removed, usually improved soon after, demonstrating a clear cause-and-effect relationship between dental health and chronic illness.

Bacteria are not the only organisms that cause problems. Our mouths are loaded with viruses, fungi, and protozoa (single-celled animals) as well. Dr. Price records a case of a woman with a huge abscess in her neck from an infected molar. Even after the tooth was extracted, the abscess persisted and resisted treatment for many weeks. A sample of the pus was taken and examined, revealing the presence of a large number of amoebas—single-celled parasites—causing the infection. Treatment for amoebas stopped the infection. Price found that amoebas were almost always found in gum disease pockets, and in at least one instance, the parasite had penetrated into the jawbone.

Dr. Price found that oral bacteria could not only spread to other areas of the body, but they also affected a patient's blood chemistry. He found that certain white blood cells decreased in number while others increased. Slight changes in the number of mature red blood cells also occurred. Hemophilia, a tendency to hemorrhage, was frequently a problem. Chronic infection caused inflammation within artery walls and raised blood pressure. Blood sugar levels increased. Alkaline reserves in the body were lowered, pushing the body towards acidosis. There was increased uric acid and nitrogen retention. Ionic calcium levels in the blood varied, becoming higher or lower than normal. All these changes caused or intensified a host of non-infectious illnesses. Heart disease, migraine headaches, diabetes, osteoporosis, hormonal imbalances, and other conditions not ordinarily associated with infections could all be influenced by dental health.

Dr. Price wasn't the only one doing this type of research. During the first three decades of the twentieth century, many other investigators performed similar studies with remarkably similar results.

Charles Mayo, M.D., the founder of the world-renowned Mayo Clinic, became interested in focal infections following years of observations made on surgical and dental patients.[9] Dr. Edward C. Rosenow was appointed to head a team of researchers at the Mayo Clinic dedicated to focal infection research. Over a 20-year period, Dr. Rosenow produced over 200 scientific papers on the subject.

Dr. Rosenow was a methodical bacteriologist who took meticulous care when performing bacterial cultures. His subsequent experiments carefully documented two important phenomenas demonstrated by the microorganisms isolated from teeth and gums: elective localization and transmutation. Elective localization is the selective preference of certain bacteria for specific locations in the body. Bacteria taken from an infected liver, for example, when injected into another animal will preferentially infect the second animal's liver. Similarly, bacteria from the mouths of patients with specific health conditions would produce similar conditions when injected into laboratory animals. For instance, Rosenow showed that streptococci isolated from the mouths of arthritis patients could cause arthritis when injected into lab animals. Streptococci from patients with gastric ulcers could be injected into dogs with the resultant induction of lesions in the stomach and gastrointestinal tract.

Bacteria from patients with cholecystitis (inflammation of the gallbladder) could induce gallbladder inflammation. These results corresponded precisely with those obtained by Dr. Price.

Dr. Rosenow's second observation, transmutation, demonstrated that certain bacteria, specifically streptococci, could change their form. By changing the conditions in which bacteria were grown in culture, such as oxygenation, sugar content, and temperature, bacteria could quickly adapt to the new environment. In the process they became smaller in size, more virulent, and their by-products became much more toxic. Aerobic organisms, which require oxygen, adapt to become anaerobic (needing no oxygen), and potentially much more destructive.

Streptococci, a common inhabitant of the mouth, have a great capability for adapting to whatever environment they encounter. This characteristic was observed soon after the introduction of antibiotics in the 1940s. Streptococci mutated, becoming immune to the drugs. Today you often see antibiotic-resistant bacteria referred to as "super germs" because they can be immune to one or several antibiotics. When streptococci end up inside the root of a tooth or migrate to the heart or joints, they can change to a more dangerous form that is likely to cause a serious infection.

In 1940, a book was published titled *Death and Dentistry* by Martin H. Fischer, M.D., a professor of physiology at the University of Cincinnati. In this book Dr. Fischer summarizes 40 years of research on focal infections. He documents associations with a wide range of illnesses including kidney disease, gallbladder disease, pneumonia, bronchitis, asthma, pleuritis, hyperthyroidism, hypothyroidism, eye infections, shingles, multiple sclerosis, senility, pharyngitis, gastritis, appendicitis, colitis, dermatitis, migraines, hypertension, and others.

Unfortunately this book, like Price's two volumes published 17 years earlier, did not get the attention it deserved. Despite the evidence

> "Like the metastasis of cancer, microorganisms from teeth and tonsils metastasize to other organs and result in similar circumstances."
>
> E.C. Rosenow, M.D.

supporting the focal infection theory, it was still only a theory. Many doctors were not convinced. They demanded further studies and more documentation.

With the introduction and mass production of penicillin in the early 1940s, and other antibiotics soon thereafter, infectious illness was thought to be a thing of the past. Infections, regardless of their origin, could be treated with antibiotics. In addition, newer, better dental techniques could repair teeth, saving them from being pulled. No longer was it acceptable to remove presumed foci of infection in the mouth. As a result, the focal theory of infection seemed to lose momentum. Teeth could be saved, and infections could easily be treated with antibiotics. The focal theory of infection fell by the wayside and was ignored, and as time passed, eventually forgotten.

RESURGENCE OF THE FOCAL INFECTION THEORY

Although ignored by both dentists and physicians for decades, the focal infection theory would not die. Too often the connection between dental health and systemic disease kept popping up. Researchers who were too young to remember the focal infection theory of earlier years rediscovered it on their own. Numerous studies began appearing in medical and dental journals connecting various acute and chronic illnesses with oral health. By the turn of the twenty-first century, the focal theory of infection had made a dramatic comeback. Today it is universally accepted, yet unfortunately, it is still underappreciated by most physicians.

The focal infection theory is now well-documented—so much so that it is no longer considered just a theory, but a fact. Today anyone who has a heart problem or an artificial joint is thought to be especially vulnerable to this type of infection and cannot undergo any dental procedure without first being treated with antibiotics.

Research over the past few years has linked oral flora to a remarkable number of health problems. Besides the most obvious infections of the jawbone, sinuses, eyes, head, and neck, some of the best-documented include heart disease, atherosclerosis (hardening of the arteries), arthritis, lung infections, osteoporosis, diabetes, and adverse pregnancy outcomes. In 2000, the U.S. Department of Health and

Human Services issued a detailed report from the Surgeon General on oral health. In this report, the connection between oral health and systemic disease was clearly outlined and documented.[10]

Although accepted by essentially all physicians and dentists, focal infections are not given as much attention as they deserve. One reason for this is that doctors feel antibiotics are an easy solution to secondary infections. Another reason is that most doctors fail to recognize the extent to which focal infections can influence overall health. Consequently, focal infections don't get much publicity. Most people have never heard about focal infections or that oral bacteria can be responsible for such things as heart attacks or strokes. When you heard this for the first time, you probably thought it sounded bizarre, and you may have had doubts.

In the following sections, evidence is presented demonstrating the connection between oral health and various common health problems.

Dental Health and Systemic Disease

In less than one minute after a dental procedure is carried out, microorganisms from the infected site may have reached the heart, lungs, and the peripheral capillary system.

People with gum disease are three times more likely to suffer a heart attack as those without gum disease.

People with periodontal disease are twice as likely to suffer from coronary artery disease as those without periodontal disease.

People with severe gum disease are twice as likely to suffer a stroke.

People with type 2 diabetes are three times more likely to develop gum disease than non-diabetic individuals.

For the skeptics who are reading this, I've also included references to a few of the hundreds of published studies, so that you may research the subject further if you desire.

Cardiovascular Health

The cardiovascular system includes the heart and blood vessels. It is cardiovascular research that has given us the most extensively documented evidence for the focal infection theory. The focal infection process is clearly seen with infective endocarditis (an infection of the heart lining and heart valves).[11-19] As far back as 1965, the *Journal of Periodontal Research* reported that 20 percent of people with existing heart problems who have dental work done, including routine tooth cleaning, develop bacterial endocarditis within several weeks after their dental visit. The infection can destroy heart valves, leading to heart failure. People with artificial heart valves are highly susceptible to infection, so they are required to take antibiotics before and after they have dental work done.

In the case of mitral valve prolapse, rheumatic heart disease, congenital heart defects, and heart murmurs, antibiotics may also be administered as a precaution whenever dental work is performed, because it is known that oral bacteria can easily attack and infect an already weakened heart.

The most common form of heart disease, and the number one cause of death worldwide, is coronary heart disease. Coronary heart disease leads to heart attacks and strokes. It occurs when plaque builds up inside arteries—the coronary artery in heart attack cases and the carotid artery in strokes. For years this condition was attributed primarily to diet and lifestyle. While diet and lifestyle undoubtedly play a part, another very important factor could be dental health.

One of the most intriguing developments in focal infection research in recent years is the association between infections and heart attacks and strokes. A large number of studies have reported associations between heart disease and chronic bacterial and viral infections. In the 1970s, researchers identified the development of atherosclerosis in the arteries of animals when they were experimentally infected with a herpes virus. In the 1980s, similar associations were reported in humans infected with a number of bacteria (e.g., *Helicobacter pylori* and

Chlamydia pneumoniae) and certain herpes viruses (particularly cytomegalovirus and HSV-1). In one study, for example, researchers at the University of Helsinki in Finland found that 27 out of 40 heart attack patients and 15 out of 30 men with heart disease carried antibodies related to chlamydia, which is more commonly known to cause gum disease and lung infections. In subjects who were free of heart disease, only 7 out of 41 had such antibodies. In another study at Baylor College of Medicine in Houston, Texas, researchers found that 70 percent of patients undergoing surgery for atherosclerosis carried antibodies to cytomegalovirus (CMV), while only 43 percent of controls did.

More evidence supporting the link between infection and cardiovascular disease showed up in the early 1990s when researchers found fragments of bacteria in arterial plaque. One of the first to discover microorganisms in atherosclerotic plaque was Brent Muhlestein, a cardiologist at the LDS Hospital in Salt Lake City and the University of Utah. Muhlestein and colleagues found evidence of chlamydia in 79 percent of plaque specimens taken from the coronary arteries of 90 heart disease patients. In comparison, fewer than four percent of normal individuals had evidence of chlamydia in artery walls.

The fact that bacteria and viruses could be involved in the development of heart disease has been a remarkable revelation. What is even more intriguing is that the organisms identified as playing a major role in heart disease don't normally take up residence in the bloodstream, but are typically found in the mouth. Could oral microbial colonies be the source? This was the next question that needed to be answered. Researchers looked at dental data and found that those people with dental infections tended to have a higher rate of heart disease and strokes.

Several studies have found that heart disease patients have more tooth decay and higher rates of gum disease than the general population. The reverse is also true. Those with poor dental health are more likely to suffer a heart attack. Subjects in these studies had their dental health evaluated and then were monitored for several years to see if those with poor dental health were more likely to get heart disease. They were.[20] For example, Robert J. Genco, D.D.S., Ph.D., of the University of Buffalo, studied 1,372 people over a 10-year period and found that heart disease was three times more prevalent for those with gum disease.[21] In the National Health and Nutritional Examination Study people with inflammation of the gums had a 25 percent increased risk of heart disease.[22] The risk was high even for those who had gum disease in the past as well as currently, indicating that gum disease may not have been completely resolved. They also found that the more severe the periodontal disease, the greater the risk of developing heart disease.

At least one out of every two adults in developed countries has antibodies to *Helicobacter pylori* (H. pylori), *Chlamydia pneumoniae*, or CMV, all of which are common inhabitants of the mouth. The presence of antibodies does not necessarily indicate an active infection or the presence of heart disease, but is a sign that infection has occurred at some time. It's common for infections from these organisms to persist indefinitely. Once infected with herpes, for example, the virus remains for life. The effectiveness of the immune system determines the degree of trouble the virus may cause. The weaker the immune system, the more likely an infection will flare up and cause problems.

When these microorganisms enter the bloodstream they can irritate the artery wall, causing chronic, low-grade infections that lack any noticeable symptoms. As microorganisms colonize the artery wall, they cause damage to arterial cells. In an effort to heal the injury, blood platelets, cholesterol, protein, and calcium combine in the artery wall, setting the stage for plaque formation.[23]

Several common species of oral bacteria, including *Steptococcus sanguis* (S. sanguis), the predominant bacterium in dental plaque, have been linked to heart disease. Bacteria that stick to teeth to form dental plaque and hardened calculus tend to do the same thing when they get into the bloodstream, but here it happens to the artery wall.

S. sanguis is found in everyone's mouth to one extent or another, depending on their oral health, and appears to play a major role in the formation of arterial plaque and blood clots. This organism can make blood sticky and induce blood clotting, which is the pivotal event in most heart attacks and stokes. The bacterium carries a surface protein called platelet aggregation association protein. This protein acts like superglue, causing blood cells to stick to each other, which causes blood to thicken and clots to form. As blood thickens, the heart must work harder to pump blood through the vessels. Blood pressure rises. As blood pressure rises, it exerts a greater force against the artery walls. This can initiate small tears in the artery wall. These injuries are patched with cholesterol, sticky blood platelets, protein, and calcium. Injuries cause inflammation. If inflammation becomes chronic due to chronic high blood pressure and/or colonization from various microbes, then cholesterol, calcium, etc. continue to accumulate, forming arterial plaque. The calcium makes plaque hard, thus the reason for the term "hardening of the arteries" in reference to arterial plaque or atherosclerosis, as it is officially termed.

As plaque builds, the opening in the artery narrows. Sticky blood has a tendency to form clots. Blood clots initiate most heart attacks and strokes by blocking arteries that feed the heart or brain. Even though arteries may be narrowed by plaque, the deposits alone are not usually enough to choke off the blood supply; the final blow is nearly always the formation of a clot that lodges itself in an already narrowed artery.

More evidence that oral bacteria are involved in the development of heart disease comes from analyzing the content of arterial plaque. Researchers have found remnants of these bacteria in 17 percent of young people and 80 percent of the elderly.[24] This shows a progression of arterial infection as we age. This makes sense since age is a risk factor for heart disease; the older we get, the more likely we will die from a heart attack or stroke. In addition, researchers have also found live oral bacteria, the smoking gun as you might say, in arterial plaque, thus demonstrating its involvement in the plaque-forming process.[25] This supplies the proof that live bacteria from the oral cavity have become inhabitants of the vessel wall. These bacteria are known to have the ability to destroy connective tissue in the mouth, suggesting that when infecting the artery wall, they may contribute to the formation of atherosclerotic plaque.

Research has further shown a correlation between the amount of periodontal bacteria in the mouth and the formation of blockages in the arteries. So, the more dental plaque and gum disease you have, the more arterial plaque you are likely to have.

The research connecting oral bacteria to heart disease is extensive.[26-32] Viruses appear to be involved as well.[33] Herpes Simplex Virus 1 (HSV-1) has been identified as one of the troublemakers. Often

Death by Toothache

Generally, dental problems such as cavities or toothaches are viewed as being trivial, although they may be painful, a visit to the dentist will quickly bring relief. Tooth decay and gum disease, however, are not trivial; they are chronic diseases. They can be the root cause for systemic infections and degenerative conditions which eventually may lead to death. Yes, death can be caused by a simple toothache. If the immune system is weak as a result of poor diet and lifestyle choices, the effects of a focal infection can be dramatic and deadly.

Rarely will a death certificate indicate that a toothache was the cause of death. The blame is usually placed on the effects of a secondary infection somewhere else in the body.

Twelve-year-old Deamonte Driver ignored the pain in one of his teeth. His mother had five children to support and at the time no job. So visiting a dentist would have to wait. Before long, the toothache was no longer noticeable. The pain seemed to have migrated into his head. The resulting headache became so unbearable that Deamonte's mother took him to the emergency room at Southern Maryland Hospital.

Deamonte's headache was caused by a brain abscess—a bacterial infection in the brain. The infection had come from the infected tooth he had complained about previously. The tooth became abscessed and the bacteria spread, causing a secondary infection in the child's brain.

Some species of streptococcus bacteria that cause tooth decay and gum disease have a tendency to accumulate in nerve tissue. From an infected tooth they can migrate up though the nerves and into the brain or spinal column, where they can cause a secondary infection. This is what happened to Deamonte.

Deamonte underwent two surgeries and the removal of the infected tooth. For several weeks afterward, he seemed to be on the mend, working with physical and occupational therapists to regain full use of his right arm and leg, which the brain infection and surgeries had impaired.

Despite thoroughly disinfecting the tooth socket and taking antibiotics, some of the infection remained and continued to spread. Within a few weeks the infection inside Deamonte's brain had returned, this time with a vengeance. Again he was rushed to the hospital, but it was too late. Deamonte died before doctors could help. The cause of Deamonte's death was attributed to a brain abscess, but the real culprit was an infected tooth.

In another case, a 57-year-old man was admitted to the hospital complaining of a toothache accompanied by a fever and swelling in his right cheek and neck. The man was a diabetic and suffered from liver cirrhosis due to excessive alcohol consumption. His immune system was obviously overworked dealing with the consequences of poor lifestyle choices. His symptoms worsened in spite of antibiotic therapy. Infection from the tooth eventually spread to his lungs (pneumonia), kidneys, and liver. After 35 days in the hospital the patient died of multi-organ failure. Antibiotics were useless. The infection in his mouth continued to feed the systemic infections until it killed him. Although weakened by other health problems, his death, like that of Deamonte's, was literally caused by an infected tooth.

Relatively young and otherwise healthy individuals are affected as well as those who are older and in poor health. A 19-year-old woman with no serious health problems had an infected tooth extracted. Soon after, she developed chest pain. Even though she was treated with antibiotics before and after the dental procedure, bacteria from the infected tooth spread to her heart. Thirteen days after the tooth extraction, she died of a heart attack brought on by the infection.

While deaths due to tooth infections are uncommon, they do happen more often than we may suspect.[99-103] In most cases, they go unreported or unrecognized, with the secondary infection getting all the blame. In most cases the patients suffered from poor nutrition, low immunity, or had other health conditions which exacerbated the situation. If a tooth infection can cause death, it can certainly cause other health problems. Even people who eat well and take care of their health can be, and are, affected by the health of their teeth.

referred to as oral herpes, it usually manifests itself as a cold sore or fever blister on the edge of the mouth. In the mouth it is relatively tame, but once it gets into the bloodstream it can become a monster (see story on page 60).

The fact that oral microbes can enter the bloodstream and spread throughout the body causing changes that affect health is firmly established. If mouth bacteria can damage the arteries and heart, then it is easy to see how they can also affect any and every other organ and tissue in the body. And they do!

Arthritis

Arthritis is characterized by inflammation and pain in the joints. It often disfigures joints and is a leading cause of disability for people over 55. There is no cure and the disease is usually progressive, but medications are used to temper symptoms. In severe cases, joint replacement is required. It generally begins when people reach middle age, but has been occurring more frequently in younger people.

Arthritis has plagued society throughout history. It is mentioned in texts from ancient Greece and Rome and evidenced in Egyptian mummies. An examination of bones, both ancient and recent, from various parts of the world show that when arthritis is present in a society, so is dental disease. For example, the ancient Egyptians suffered from many of the same diseases as we do—arthritis, atherosclerosis, and gum disease. Worn teeth, cavities, and evidence of abscesses testify to the poor dental health of some Egyptians. Interestingly, in populations where dental health was good and cavities rare, arthritis, as well as atherosclerosis and other common degenerative diseases, was also rare or non-existent.

One of the most often reported results of treating dental disease is the effect on arthritis. When infected teeth are pulled, arthritic symptoms soon disappear. The connection was noticed in the seventh century BC by the ancient Assyrians. Three hundred years later Hippocrates noted the connection as well. During the early nineteenth century Dr. Benjamin Rush, a Pennsylvanian doctor and signer of the Declaration of Independence, reported that arthritis went away in some of his patients after they had infected teeth extracted. In the late 1800s and early 1900s, the same phenomenon was reported by dentists, and papers were written about this relationship in the medical journals of the day. Even now, patients will sometimes mention to their dentists the relief of arthritis after receiving dental treatment.[34] However, most patients never discuss this with their dentists because arthritis is not ordinarily considered a dental concern, so there seems no need to mention it. Since recovery occurs weeks after dental work, many patients don't even make the connection.

The first modern medical papers published linking chronic focal infection to arthritis appeared in the late nineteenth and early twentieth centuries.[35-39] Dr. Weston A. Price's monumental work published in the 1920s also supported the link. Dr. Price reported numerous cases where patients gained relief from arthritis after having infected teeth removed and the development of arthritis in rabbits when these same teeth were surgically inserted under their skin.

More recently, a number of studies have demonstrated that oral bacteria can cause or trigger arthritis.[40-42] Researchers Lens and Beertsen, performed experiments similar to those of Weston A. Price.[43] Instead of injecting teeth or bacteria under the skin of lab animals as Price did, Lens and Beertsen injected antigens into the gums of the animals. This actually represents more accurately how a substance located in the gums, like an infected tooth, could affect the animal's health. The result was the production of knee joint inflammation.

Mouth bacteria, once they get into the bloodstream, tend to collect and cause infection in the weakest areas of the body. Certain bacteria apparently have an affinity for the joints. Joints that have already been weakened by disease or trauma are primary locations for secondary infection. Limbs or joints that are replaced by artificial joints and prostheses also appear to be prime targets for infection. Mouth bacteria readily attack these locations.[44-47] For this reason, antibiotics are routinely given to patients with such problems before and after any dental procedure.

Lung and Bronchial Infections

Pulling out all your teeth may be good for your lungs. Why? It has been observed that certain lung infections are rare in those people who don't have any teeth.[48] I don't necessarily recommend that you pull all of your teeth, but several studies have demonstrated an association between oral health and respiratory diseases such as pneumonia and chronic obstructive pulmonary disease.[49-52] Chronic obstructive pulmonary disease refers to a group of slowly progressive diseases of the airways that are characterized by a gradual loss of lung function. This group includes emphysema, chronic bronchitis, and asthma.

A connection between the mouth and the lungs isn't too surprising. If the mouth is full of bacteria, it is only reasonable to assume that some of it ends up in our lungs. Of course, if we have a lot of the wrong types of bacteria in our mouths, they may cause trouble in our lungs and airways.

Bacteria that inhabit the mouth are often found causing trouble in the bronchial tubes and lungs. *Streptococcus pneumoniae*, a frequent oral troublemaker, is a common cause of bacterial pneumonia. Chlamydia, mycoplasma, and neisseria are other oral bacteria that can cause pneumonia. While these bacteria are often in our mouths and airways, they don't always cause trouble. Normally, the body's immune system fights off these troublemakers. But in times of excessive stress, malnutrition, or other infections, the immune system's resistance is depressed, and these organisms can quickly get out of hand. When a person's resistance is lowered, bacteria work their way into the lungs and inflame the air sacs. The lungs fill with fluid, preventing the delivery of oxygen into the bloodstream. This is what happens when someone gets pneumonia. Pneumonia is a common illness affecting all age groups and is a leading cause of death among the elderly or those who are chronically ill.

Asthma is another common respiratory problem. It is a chronic disease that affects the airways carrying air in and out of the lungs. These airways occasionally constrict, become inflamed, and fill with excessive amounts of mucus, making breathing very difficult. For reasons not known, asthma is increasing in Western populations. It is generally believed to be incurable.

In recent years, a growing body of evidence suggests that the most severe forms of asthma are caused by infections. Where do the infections come from? You guessed it—the mouth! The primary guilty party appears to be *Chlaymdia pneumoniae*, a microbe that is a common cause of pneumonia.[53]

In asthma, bacteria infect the airways leading to the lungs. The bacteria cling to mucous membranes causing irritation and chronic low-grade inflammation. This has led researchers to propose treating asthma with antibiotics. Clinical studies using this approach have proven to be surprisingly effective.[54]

Many people can attest to the use of antibiotic therapy to "cure" asthma. "My story is proof that extremely severe asthma can be cured," says Jim Quinlan. "I came close to dying when a near fatal asthma attack put me into full respiratory and cardiac arrest!"

As with many asthma sufferers, Jim's flare-ups were intense and sleeping was difficult. "Every single night was hell for me. I spent many evenings in hospital emergency rooms because my asthma was completely out of control…The only relief I ever had was when I took a dose pack of steroids. I had air cleaners in my bedroom, a humidifier by my bedside, special electronic air cleaners on our furnace, a breathing machine with a bunch of tubes at my bedside (one that delivers misted medicine). My bedroom looked like a hospital ward. Despite all the gizmos, I still could not breathe during the night and would cough so much that my neighbors could hear me hacking and coughing, even when all the windows were closed."

A pharmacist friend told Jim about some new research connecting asthma with bacteria. Jim found a doctor who was willing to treat him with antibiotics. It was discouraging at first. It took him six months and several rounds of antibiotics before he no longer needed an inhaler. It was nearly a year before he felt completely normal.

"Now that my asthma is completely cured, I live an active lifestyle that includes walking on the beaches and hiking on the Florida trails and parks. I've backpacked hundreds of miles of the Appalachian trail and also waded/slogged through 40 miles of Everglades swamps in deep mud and water up to waist deep. I did these hikes with no inhalers, no medicines, and best of all, no asthma."

Preliminary research has shown that bacteria are responsible for up to 60 percent of all cases of asthma, and it may even be higher. In such cases antibiotics may be useful, but as in Jim's case, it took time. If the infection is coming from a tooth, antibiotics aren't always as effective as they are for other infections because bacteria can burrow inside teeth where antibiotics can't easily reach. Fortunately, Jim was persistent enough to continue with treatment until he got results.

Pregnancy Complications

Gum disease not only affects you, but may also affect your unborn child. It is remarkable how oral health can affect nearly every facet of our lives. Fetal development is another condition that can be directly influenced by the health of our mouths.

It has been observed that periodontal disease can adversely affect pregnancy outcome, increasing the risk of delivering preterm and low birth weight babies. Mothers of preterm and low birth weight babies have a significantly greater incidence of periodontal disease.[55-58] Research shows that pregnant women with periodontal disease are seven and a half times more likely to have a premature or underweight delivery and the more severe the disease, the greater effect it has on the baby.[59]

Low birth weight is considered 5.5 pounds (2,500 g) or less. The birth weight of an infant isn't just about size; it has a significant impact on the baby's health. An infant's birth weight is the most potent single indicator of the infant's future health status. A low birth weight baby has a statistically greater chance than a normal weight baby of developing diseases and of dying early in life. About one in every 13 infants born in the US is a low birth weight infant, and about one-fourth of those die within the first month of life.

How does oral bacteria affect a developing fetus? Studies show that bacteria commonly found in the mouth and associated with periodontal diseases can find their way into the amniotic fluid of pregnant women.[60] Amniotic fluid is a liquid that surrounds an unborn baby during pregnancy. Any contamination of the amniotic fluid, such as a bacteria, could potentially be dangerous to both the mother and baby.

Another problem linked to oral health that can occur during pregnancy is preeclampsia.[61] This is a serious condition that occurs during the second half of pregnancy. It is characterized by high blood pressure and water retention. Additional symptoms may include headache, nausea, vomiting, abdominal pain, and visual disturbances. Preeclampsia occurs in about one out of every 20 pregnancies. Untreated it may develop into eclampsia, a life-threatening form of

Pregnancy and Fetal Development

Pregnant women with poor dental health are seven and a half times more likely to deliver prematurely.

The human body produces a total of 52 primary and permanent teeth. Of this number, 32 begin during fetal development. We have 20 primary (baby) teeth and 32 permanent teeth.

Vitamin deficiency during pregnancy can affect an infant's tooth development causing imperfections in the teeth, distortions in the bridge of the mouth, and misalignment of the teeth, increasing the child's susceptibility to dental problems.

toxemia that can cause severe convulsions, kidney failure, and even death for mother or fetus.

In three clinical studies, researchers at Tulane University in New Orleans determined that dental treatment led to a 57 percent reduction of low birth weight deliveries, and a 50 percent reduction in preterm births.

It is estimated that 60-75 percent of pregnant women have gingivitis. Women who are pregnant or are considering becoming pregnant, should pay particular attention to their dental health to assure that they and their babies have the best health possible.

Gastrointestinal Health

While troublesome microbes in the mouth usually spread to other parts of the body by way of the bloodstream, they can also enter the body in other ways. Just as mouth organisms can travel through your windpipe into your lungs, they can also go down the esophagus and into the digestive tract. We are continually swallowing the microbes that flourish in our mouths. Ordinarily they pose little threat because the hydrochloric acid and digestive enzymes in the stomach make short work of them. However, not all of them are killed. Many manage to survive and are passed along into the intestinal tract. This is how most of the microbes in the intestines and colon got there in the first place. Most of these microbes do us no harm and are happy to live in the digestive tract. You may be surprised to learn that potentially harmful organisms such as E. coli and *Candida albicans* also enter the intestinal tract through the mouth. E. coli and candida are commonly found in the mouth to one extent or another.

Candida is a single-celled fungus, or yeast, which inhabits the entire gastrointestinal tract. Localized candida infections can occur anywhere along the digestive tract, as well as on or near other mucus membranes. Thrush, a common illness in infants, is an overgrowth of oral candida. Diaper rash is also caused by candida, as are vaginal yeast infections. Flare-ups often occur after taking antibiotics, which kill bacteria but have no effect on fungus. Without competition from bacteria the yeast multiply rapidly, causing localized and systemic yeast infections.

H. pylori is another inhabitant of the mouth that can cause gastrointestinal troubles. H. pylori often accompanies other bacteria as part of the plaque buildup on teeth. It can migrate to the stomach, where it eats small holes in the stomach's lining, producing painful ulcers, and may also cause stomach cancer.[62-63] H. pylori causes about 90 percent of stomach ulcers. Although most of us have H. pylori living in our mouths, most of us do not have stomach ulcers. If your stomach is healthy, H. pylori poses little threat. The regular use of certain drugs, medications, and foods can affect the environment of the stomach. Pain relievers (aspirin, Advil, Motrin, Aleve, etc.) reduce a key substance that helps preserve the protective lining of your stomach. Antacids lower the acidity level of the stomach, allowing bacteria to survive long enough to burrow into the wall of the stomach or pass into the intestinal tract. Excessive alcohol use can irritate and erode your stomach lining, which makes your stomach more vulnerable to attack by harmful microbes. Stress, malnutrition, and illness can all lower immunity, increasing susceptibility to H. pylori infection.

Microorganisms from periodontal lesions have also been implicated in the pathogenesis of inflammatory bowel diseases (IBD) such as Crohn's disease and ulcerative colitis.[64] Although the cause of IBD is still unknown, bacteria or viruses have been suggested as likely suspects. Evidence for the involvement of streptococci was given by Dr. Weston A. Price and again in 1939 by Milton J. Rosenau, M.D., professor of Preventive Medicine and Hygiene at Harvard Medical School (not to be confused with Dr. Edward C. Rosenow of the Mayo Clinic discussed earlier). In an article published in the *Journal of the American Dental Association*, Dr. Rosenau reported isolating streptococci bacteria from an ulcer in the bowel of a patient who was suffering with colitis. He injected the bacteria into several animals, reproducing the colitis. The source of the patient's bowel infection was traced to a crowned bicuspid which had a large abscess at its root end. Cultures were then made from the abscess and planted in some of the teeth of a dog. X-ray photographs revealed these teeth developed abscesses similar to those found in the patient. After 16 months, the dog developed ulcerative colitis. Streptococcus is a normal inhabitant of the mouth and digestive tract, yet inside a tooth it can mutate. In its mutated form it can migrate to other parts of the body such as the gastrointestinal tract where it apparently can cause ulcerations. Since streptococcus is commonly found in the gut, it is generally overlooked as a cause of IBD.

More recently, it has been found that those people with IBD appear to have unusual microorganisms colonizing their oral cavity that apparently may also play a role in the development of the disease. One of these organisms is the small, mobile bacteria *Wolinella succinogenes*.

Until recently wolinella was considered to be harmless because it is a normal inhabitant of the digestive tract of cows, where it appears

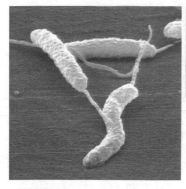
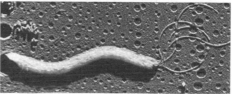

The bacteria in your mouth can influence the health of your entire digestive tract. Two potential troublemakers: wolinella (left) and H. pylori (above).

to cause no harm. Genetically it is related to two microbes that cause stomach disorders in humans: H. pylori and *Campylobacter jejuni*. In humans wolinella displays much of the same virulence exhibited by H. pylori. In the mouth wolinella usually settles in the space between the teeth and gums and in dental root canal infections.

The cause of Crohn's disease, colitis, and other irritable bowel syndromes has been a mystery to medical science. We now have a couple of possible suspects, which were, until recently, thought to be harmless. You can compare the current state of knowledge to the one that existed a decade ago for stomach ulcers. Many doctors at that time rejected the idea that bacteria, rather than stress or diet, might be the cause, but the theory was ultimately proven correct, and now most ulcers are treated with antibiotics.

Osteoporosis

Bones, like any other organ in the body, are living tissues. They are not like cement blocks that don't change once they are made. You can think of the skeleton like a house that is continually being remodeled. As living tissue, new bone cells are continually being formed while others are dismantled. This is why broken bones can grow back together and why athletes develop strong, dense bones. When we are young, new bone cells are produced faster than the old ones are torn down. As we grow older, bone absorption outpaces bone formation. Over time, our bones gradually become more porous and weaker.

The process of bone production and reabsorption is regulated by a variety of factors, including hormones and cytokines. Cytokines are substances that are produced by the cells of our immune system in order to stimulate inflammation. Inflammation is needed to fight off infection. Unfortunately, inflammation near bone tissue stimulates bone reabsorption, resulting in net bone loss.

Periodontal disease has long been associated with bone loss. Infected teeth cause inflammation that often weakens the jaw bone. The bone holding teeth in place begins to dissolve and teeth become loose. When bacteria or their toxins enter the bloodstream, the immune system responds to the invasion by producing cytokines that stimulate inflammation. If the infection is chronic, inflammation becomes chronic. If the infection is isolated to certain areas of the body like the jaw, skull, or hips, localized degradation of the bone occurs, as seen in Paget's disease.[65] If the infection is systemic, bone density throughout the body can decline.[66] In this way, periodontal disease can lead to or exacerbate osteoporosis.[67-68] Both periodontal disease and osteoporosis are common problems among the elderly. Osteoporosis is more common among woman than men. Changes in hormone levels during menopause often affect the bacterial colonies in the mouth, which may in turn increase systemic inflammation, accelerating bone loss.

Diabetes

As odd as it may seem, diabetes can also be affected by oral health. Diabetes is not caused by an infection, but occurs as a result of poor blood sugar regulation. After eating, much of the food we consume is converted into glucose and released into the bloodstream. Glucose is also known as blood sugar. Our cells use glucose as food to produce energy.

Glucose, however, cannot simply enter the cells. The hormone insulin is needed to shuttle glucose from the bloodstream into the cells. As blood sugar levels rise after a meal, more insulin is released to maintain normal glucose levels. As blood sugar levels drop, insulin levels also fall. In this way blood sugar levels are maintained within a narrow range.

In type 2 diabetes (by far the most common form of diabetes) the cells have become desensitized to the action of insulin. This is called insulin resistance. Glucose transport into cells occurs much slower than normal. This causes blood sugar levels to rise above normal and remain elevated for an extended amount of time. Too much sugar has serious consequences, potentially leading to diabetes-induced coma and even death. So keeping blood sugar levels under control is important for diabetics.

Insulin resistance is a key factor in the development of type 2 diabetes. There appear to be many things that work together to promote insulin resistance, but the major contributing factor is believed to be proinflammatory cytokines. When bacteria and their toxins enter the bloodstream from infected teeth, they trigger the immune system to release cytokines that generate inflammation. Chronic systemic inflammation desensitizes the insulin receptors on the cells, causing insulin resistance, which leads to elevated blood sugar. Proinflammatory cytokines can also damage pancreatic cells that produce insulin, thus reducing the body's ability to produce insulin, degrading blood sugar control even more.

Over 200 studies have been published in medical journals in recent years describing the relationship between diabetes and periodontal disease. From these studies it is evident that periodontal disease can cause or exacerbate insulin resistance.[69-72] Diabetics are twice as likely to have a periodontal infection as non-diabetics.

Studies also show that treating periodontal disease can significantly improve insulin resistance and improve blood sugar control in diabetics.[73] Some researchers believe that chronic periodontal disease can even cause diabetes.[74-75] Consequently, dentists are encouraged to treat their diabetic patients with care so as not to exacerbate their condition by invasive dental procedures. This is not to say that all cases of diabetes are caused by dental problems, but it does show that poor dental health can contribute to diabetes, and healthy teeth reduce the risk and improve blood sugar control.

Diet has a definite influence on diabetes. The worst foods a diabetic can consume are sugar and refined carbohydrates. Not only do they raise blood sugar levels, but they also encourage the growth of troublesome mouth bacteria that cause infection and inflammation, which promotes insulin resistance. These foods also promote obesity, another risk factor for diabetes.

Nervous System

The nervous system comprises the brain, spinal cord, and nerves. Oral bacteria often find their way into nerve tissue. Certain viruses, such as the herpes virus, after initial infection take up residence in nerve tissue, where the infection often remains dormant except for periodic flare-ups during times of stress or compromised immunity.

Oral bacteria traveling though the nerves may end up in the brain, where an infection results. A tooth abscess can precipitate a brain abscess.[76-78]

Meningitis occurs when bacteria or viruses enter the spinal fluid and infect the membranes surrounding the brain and spinal cord. It is a serious, sometimes fatal, illness that can cause headaches, fever, vomiting, and stiff neck. Meningitis can be caused by organisms from a variety of sources, including the mouth.[79-81]

If oral flora can travel through the nerves to the brain and spinal cord, then they can affect just about any nerve tissue throughout the body. Indeed, oral bacteria have been found to cause infections in nerve cells throughout the body.[82-83]

If the immune system is strong enough it can keep serious infections in nerve and brain tissue at bay. However, a continual stream of bacteria into these tissues can cause chronic inflammation. There may be no symptoms immediately noticeable, but over time the inflammation damages nerve tissue. Several studies have identified correlations between neurological degeneration such as Alzheimer's disease, Parkinson's disease, and multiple sclerosis with poor dental health.[84-86] For instance, in one study 144 participants between the ages of 75 and 98 were studied over a period of several years. Their dental as well as mental health was monitored. Autopsies of 118 participants who died during the study were also available. Researchers found that the greater the number of teeth missing, due to tooth decay and gum disease, the higher the incidence of dementia and Alzheimer's disease.[87]

One in ten persons over the age of 65 and as many as half the population aged 85 and over have Alzheimer's disease. Will you be one of them? Poor dental health is now recognized as a risk factor for Alzheimer's disease. So taking good care of your teeth can also help you take good care of your mind. Brushing the teeth is not sufficient, as all the people in these studies brushed their teeth regularly and it didn't prevent the disease. However, oil pulling can help. It's a simple procedure that can help prevent a potentially devastating condition.

Infectious and Chronic Disease

Once bacteria, viruses, fungi, and protozoa from the mouth enter the bloodstream they can end up anywhere in the body, causing infection in any tissue or organ. Usually these organisms or their toxic waste products collect in the weakest parts of our bodies, where they can cause irritation and disease. Your painful joints, low back pain, kidney or liver problems may be the work of microscopic invaders. Our primary defense is the immune system.

DR. G MEDICAL EXAMINER

Dr. Jan Garavaglia (a.k.a. Dr. G) is a medical examiner (coroner) in Orlando, Florida. As a medical examiner, her job is to determine the cause of death of individuals who die unexpectedly or under unusual circumstances. She has a cable network program—*Dr. G: Medical Examiner*—that airs on the Discovery Health Channel. The program highlights some of her more interesting cases.

In one episode, a woman in her 20s, complaining of various symptoms, was admitted to the hospital. She was given antibiotics, but her condition worsened and she began to develop small lesions all over her body. It appeared that she had a simple case of chicken pox. Two days later, however, she was dead. Chicken pox isn't normally a life-threatening condition; something else was involved. Her body was sent to Dr. G to determine the cause of death.

Dr. G performed a detailed autopsy. When she opened the body, she found that the woman's internal organs were also riddled with lesions. The woman's liver was so badly pitted it was determined that she died from liver failure. What caused the lesions that attacked her body and destroyed her liver? That was Dr. G's next challenge.

Chicken pox was the first suspect, but it appeared that there was another, more virulent, entity involved. Dr. G took tissue samples of the lesions on the woman's skin and liver and sent them to the lab for examination. When the lab results came back Dr. G was shocked. It was a common form of herpes—herpes simplex virus 1 (HSV-1). HSV-1 is usually confined to the mouth and rarely spreads to other parts of the body.

HSV-1 is common; by the age of 50 some 50-80 percent of the population is infected. Once you get the virus, you have it for life. Normally, it doesn't cause too much trouble. It usually makes its presence known by producing "cold sores" or "fever blisters" on the lips. The immune system usually keeps the infection under control. Only when the immune system is compromised do flare-ups occur.

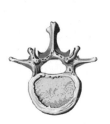

So why did this patient have such a violent case of herpes? Dr. G's explanation was that her immune system must have been so weak that it allowed the virus to spread. What weakened her immune system? It certainly wasn't age, as she was in the prime of life. Dr. G's first guess was HIV—the AIDS virus. Secondary infections like herpes are often the cause of death in HIV infected individuals. But the woman's blood tested negative to HIV. Dr. G couldn't find an answer. The case was closed.

There is an answer. Although Dr. G. noted the presence of oral herpes, she failed to look at the patient's mouth in detail and examine her teeth and gums. It is highly probable that the young woman had gum disease. Bacteria entering her bloodstream through the diseased gums were slowly poisoning her body. Her immune system was working overtime fighting off the constant invasion of bacteria. When her herpes flared up, the virus wasn't confined to her mouth, as it usually is. It, too, passed through the bleeding gums and entered the bloodstream, where it was carried throughout the body. In her body, this relatively harmless virus became deadly.

Any type of bacteria, virus, fungi, or parasite, no matter how benign it may appear, can become deadly when it enters the bloodstream. Good bacteria that help fight off harmful bacteria in the mouth or gut can become villainous when removed from their normal environment. For this reason, it is essential that teeth and gums be healthy.

If you are healthy and your immune system is functioning as it should, these troublemakers are kept in check and don't cause too much of a problem. However, if you have periodontal disease and tooth decay, you are cultivating a breeding ground for harmful bacteria that continually enter your bloodstream. Consequently, your immune system is constantly fighting a battle with an endless stream of invaders. Combine this with stress from daily life, poor dietary habits, poor lifestyle choices, drug, tobacco, and alcohol use, or other factors, and your immune system can be so overwhelmed that it cannot adequately fight off infection.

One of the first responses the immune system has to infection is the production of cytokines that stimulate inflammation. In the short run, inflammation is beneficial and aids in the fight against the infection. However, if the infection is chronic, inflammation also becomes chronic. Inflammation is meant to be a temporary defensive tactic to quickly rid the body of invading organisms. Inflammation causes many chemical changes that in the short run are essentially harmless, but can be destructive to tissues and cells if inflammation becomes chronic. Most of the conditions we classify as degenerative disease involve chronic inflammation, and much of the pain and damage associated with these conditions are a result of the inflammation. As mentioned earlier in this chapter, chronic inflammation can alter blood chemistry, which can cause or trigger any number of disease conditions. Consequently, virtually any chronic health problem could be caused or at least intensified by oral infections, including various forms of cancer, insomnia, migraine headaches, kidney dysfunction, lupus, hormonal disturbances, chronic fatigue, multiple sclerosis, psoriasis, allergies, visual problems, gallbladder disease, liver disease, infertility—the list is endless. More and more studies are being published linking these and other conditions to oral infections.[88-97]

With all this said, it must be emphasized that not all cases of heart disease, asthma, osteoporosis or any of the conditions described in this chapter result from oral infections. Most of these conditions can have multiple causes. Oral infections are just one of the possible causes or contributing factors. However, as more evidence surfaces, it is becoming clear that oral health exerts a significant and generally unrecognized influence on our overall health.

So, if infections from the mouth cause or contribute to so many health problems, why can't all these conditions simply be treated with antibiotics? That seems like a logical approach, and that is the path taken by most doctors. However, if the problem stems from an infected tooth, antibiotics don't always work.[98] Antibiotics may kill the bacteria in various parts of the body, but the infected tooth may remain infected and continue to leak bacteria and toxins into the bloodstream. So after a course of antibiotics has quieted a systemic infection, new bacteria from the infected tooth keep the fire alive and the problem will eventually resurface.

Antibiotics cannot always reach the deep-seated infections located inside teeth or buried deep in the gums. Even if the bacteria were killed, the mouth continues to collect and breed more bacteria. It is never sterile.

You would have to take antibiotics continually to keep infectious microbes under control but that isn't a good idea. The most troublesome bacteria are highly adaptable and can easily become resistant to antibiotics, rendering the drugs useless. In addition, drugs, including antibiotics, all carry risks and can have adverse side effects that can create more problems than they solve.

Another major limitation with antibiotics is that they are useful only for bacteria; they can't do a thing to viruses, fungi, or protozoa, which also cause systemic infections. In fact, antibiotics can increase the risk of infection from these other organisms. Except for an acute infection, antibiotic treatment for oral bacteria is impractical.

After reading this chapter you can see how important oral health is to whole-body health. The obvious solution to having a healthy smile and a healthy body is by maintaining good oral hygiene. Despite brushing, flossing, using disinfectant mouthwashes, and getting regular dental checkups, most of us still suffer from some level of dental decay or gum disease. There is a solution—a very simple solution. The answer is Oil Pulling Therapy.

Chapter 4

Deadly Dentistry

Your dentist may have more influence on your overall health than any other health care practitioner. He or she can save you from a myriad of infectious and degenerative diseases, or can be the cause of them.

As you have learned in this book, the health of your mouth can have a direct influence on the health of your entire body. Keeping your teeth and gums healthy can protect you from disease. For this reason, it is wise to visit your dentist for regular check-ups and cleaning, if necessary. You don't want an infection to take hold and grow into a bigger problem. While proper oral hygiene can reduce the need for regular dental checkups, if you do develop a problem, you should not ignore it. A serious problem is not likely to go away on its own.

On the other side of the coin, dentists can also be the cause of many of our health problems. Many dental procedures, while improving our smile, may lead to serious health problem later on. What a dentist puts into your mouth, or doesn't put in, can have a marked influence on your health. Cosmetic appearance should not be your sole criteria for having dental work done, since some procedures increase health risks. Knowing the consequences of these dental procedures will empower you with the knowledge to make informed decisions in regard to your dental care.

ROOT CANALS

When Dr. Weston A. Price was doing his research on the relationship between dental health and systemic disease, much of his work involved root canals. Root canalled teeth extracted from ill patients and implanted into rabbits caused similar diseases in the animals. It became obvious that bacteria survived the disinfecting process during root canal treatment, leaving infection present. The infections often went unnoticed.

Price experimented with different disinfecting agents, yet none were able to completely rid root canalled teeth of bacteria. *All* root canalled teeth remained infected and, therefore, had the potential to cause local and systemic infections.

Since the 1920s when Price first published his findings, root canal procedures have greatly increased. Today, approximately 40 million root canal treatments are performed in the U.S. alone each year. At this rate, if each person in the country were to receive one root canal, every man, woman, and child would have a root canal within seven and a half years. Obviously, some people have no root canals and others have many. Since a tooth must be badly rotted in order to need a root canal, these figures illustrate the generally poor dental health of the populace. Despite pearly white teeth, dental decay is a major problem. Cosmetic appearance doesn't always reflect dental health.

One of the arguments favoring root canals is that procedures have improved over the years. Strong disinfectants are used and teeth are thoroughly cleaned so that there is little risk of infection nowadays. Although procedures may have improved, the underlying problem with root canals still exists.

The problem lies in the structure of the tooth. Bacteria that cause most root canal infections are not on the surface of the tooth, or even inside the root canal, but come from inside the tooth itself. Although teeth look like they are dense and solid, they are, in fact, very porous. Dentin, which makes up most of the structure of teeth, is composed of millions of microscopic tubes called tubules. These tubules are so numerous that if those contained in a single small front tooth were placed end to end, they would extend for three miles. Tubules exist as passageways to bring nutrients from the root and bloodstream to the

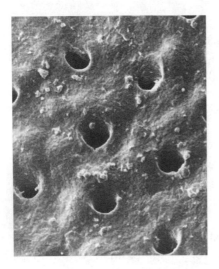

Microscopic view of tubules in the dentin of a human tooth.

living tooth. Even the hard enamel covering the top of the tooth is porous enough to permit movement of this fluid.

Bacteria often enter the tubules, particularly if the tooth has been attacked by decay. This is especially true for badly decayed teeth that are candidates for root canals. Once bacteria penetrate deep into the tubules, they can remain indefinitely. Antibiotics and disinfectants have no power over them. Burrowed deep inside the tubules, drugs and disinfectants are unable to reach them. Bacteria have a safe haven where they flourish and multiply. No matter how well the dentist cleans and disinfects a root canalled tooth, it will *always* harbor bacteria. Therefore, *all* root canalled teeth are potential breeding grounds for bacteria.

Dr. Price tried soaking infected teeth in powerful disinfectants, thoroughly killing all surface bacteria, yet when the teeth were inserted into animals, infections still occurred. A dentist can't come close to disinfecting a tooth this thoroughly while it is still in the patient's mouth, thus demonstrating the fact that no tooth can be completely bacteria-free regardless of the treatment it has received.

George E. Meinig, D.D.S., one of the founding members of the American Association of Endodontists (root canal specialists), and author of *Root Canal Cover-Up*, says, "Root canal materials and treatment have greatly improved over the years, but the underlying problem still

66

exists: bacteria are live inside the tooth. Antibiotics and disinfectants do not get rid of them. No root canalled tooth is free from potentially harmful bacteria. It is safer to pull a severely diseased tooth rather than plug and cap it, forming a breeding ground of decay, sealing in poisons and bacteria that will leak into the bloodstream for the rest of your life."

A root-filled tooth may not be painful or show any noticeable signs of infection, even on x-rays. "Every dentist knows x-ray pictures do not accurately reveal infection which can be present in teeth," says Dr. Meinig. "Dentists who extract teeth often find root canal filled teeth have infection and pus around them—even when they look fine. Some have turned black and others smell very bad. Endodontists rarely perform extractions, so they are not aware of these signs of root canal treatment failure."

Not all people who have root-filled teeth experience problems. Dr. Price found that those who didn't have problems had remarkably good immune systems and were able to control the bacteria and prevent infection. However, he also found that when these people had an accident, came down with the flu, or suffered from some stressful

---

It Started With A Root Canal

"I had a root canal when I was in my 30's. I kept telling the dentist that it hurt but no dentist would believe me. When I was about 55, I went to a new dentist and said I wanted the tooth pulled. He did, and a river of pus ran down my chin. The next day, the tooth next to the pulled tooth started to die. That tooth had to be pulled. Years later, I had another tooth die. All these teeth were in the same area. I went to several dentists and all of them said "root canal," but I said "no way." I wanted to know why my teeth were dying and all in the same area. Well I finally found out I had an infection in my jaw. I found a dentist and he pulled several of my teeth on one side. My jaw was infected from the first root canal. My bone was like soup."

Alice W.

event, the overburdened immune system allowed infection to occur, eventually leading to the development of rheumatism, arthritis, heart problems, and other secondary conditions. Even the natural process of aging reduces the effectiveness of the immune system. A younger person may not experience any serious effects from root canals, but as he or she ages the likelihood increases. Many of those aches and pains and symptoms of "aging" may really be the consequence of root canals.

One of the benefits of my Oil Pulling Therapy is that it can help prevent infections that lead to tooth decay. In many cases active infections can be eliminated and teeth saved. However, if decay is advanced, it may be too late to save the teeth. Your dentist may recommend a root canal and assure you it is completely safe. After reading this book you are more informed than most patients and can make an informed decision.

Sometimes it may be best to have a root canal. If you are already missing one or more molars near a root-filled tooth or a tooth that is a candidate for a root canal, removing another molar can make chewing difficult. Eating fresh vegetables and high fiber foods may not be possible. If your immune system is strong, you may want to keep a root canalled tooth in place so that you can continue eating healthfully. If you don't plan to eat healthfully, however, you might as well get the tooth pulled.

Having a tooth pulled is an important decision. If you are doubtful about taking that step, I suggest reading Dr. Meinig's book *Root Canal Cover-Up*.

AMALGAM FILLINGS

One of baseball's greatest players was New York Yankee first baseman Lou Gehrig. Gehrig was a power hitter second only to teammate Babe Ruth. He spent 13 years with the Yankees playing in 2,130 consecutive games. He never missed a game due to sickness or injury. His great strength and endurance earned him the nickname of "The Iron Horse." Despite his athletic powers, Gehrig's career was cut short by a rare neurological disease which forced him to retire at the relatively young age of 36. Two years later, in 1941, he was dead.

Today, amyotrophic lateral sclerosis (ALS), commonly known as Lou Gehrig's Disease, affects some 30,000 people in the US and about

2 per 100,000 individuals worldwide. It is an autoimmune disease that is characterized by deterioration of nerve cells and loss of muscle control.

How can a relatively young, otherwise healthy individual like Gehrig, succumb to such a devastating degenerative disease? Doctors don't know what causes it. There are some theories, one of which is chemical or heavy metal poisoning, with mercury being the primary suspect.

Unlike other metals, mercury is a liquid, which makes it useful for many industrial purposes. Mercury has long been known as a deadly poison. In fact, it is one of the most toxic substances known to science. Just breathing in the vapor that naturally emits from the mercury can cause disease and death. Throughout history it was commonly used as a disinfectant and pesticide. Mine workers exposed to mercury vapor suffered many neurological problems and had unusually short lives. In the hat industry of the eighteenth and nineteenth centuries, "hatters" used mercuric nitrate paste to prevent mold from growing on the hats. Inhalation of the mercury vapors sent many of them to the madhouse, leading to the saying "he is as mad as a hatter."

In more recent years the industrial use of mercury has created environmental problems. One of the most well-known occurred in Minamata, Japan in the 1950s and early 1960s. People were becoming sick with an unknown illness. Both adults and infants were affected. The symptoms included progressive blindness, deafness, loss of coordination, and intellectual deterioration. Nearly half of all the cases reported ended in death. Ultimately, the cause was discovered to be methylmercury poisoning and was traced to the consumption of contaminated fish. Industrial waste was being dumped into the bay where these people fished. The fish accumulated the mercury in their bodies. Some of these people where eating the fish every day. Infants who contracted the disease had not eaten any fish, but their mothers had, and even though the mothers may not have exhibited any symptoms during their pregnancies, the poison had been affecting their unborn babies. Regardless of where you live, today we are often warned about the dangers of eating fish because of possible mercury contamination.

Although it is not known if Lou Gehrig's condition was a result of mercury poisoning, it is highly possible. Where did he get exposure to mercury? The most likely source was his dental fillings. As remarkable as it may appear, his dental work may have been the cause of his demise.

Metal or "silver" fillings used in dentistry are composed of a combination of silver, tin, zinc, copper, and mercury. They are referred to as amalgam fillings. Silver, tin, zinc, and copper make up 50 percent of the amalgam with mercury comprising the remaining fifty percent. There is actually very little silver in amalgams. They more accurately should be called mercury fillings, but silver has a much less menacing sound.

Why in the world would dentists purposely put mercury, a deadly poison, into someone's mouth? Common sense would make you wonder. The reason boils down to functionality. Mercury amalgams make good plugs for holes in decayed teeth. Preserving the health of the patient doesn't have anything to do with it.

Before the invention of mercury amalgams in 1819, the only other practical option was gold foil. Gold, however, was expensive. Other metal alloys were tried but in order to put them into a tooth, they had to be melted and pored in hot. This didn't sit well with most patients. Mercury is liquid and when it is combined with other metals like copper and silver, it makes the alloy pliable enough to be molded into a cavity. After it has been set in the tooth, it gradually hardens, making it ideal for fillings. After nearly 200 years, mercury fillings are still used by dentists.

Even in the early 1800s amalgam fillings were controversial. Mercury was recognized as a potent poison. Some dentists objected to the use of amalgams, but other than gold leaf, there was no other practical alternative. Many patients could not afford gold fillings and amalgams were their only option. The debate raged on. The American Society of Dental Surgeons deemed the use of mercury fillings to be unethical and forbid its members from using it. Members were obliged to sign pledges promising not to use amalgam upon threat of expulsion from the association. A large number of practicing dentists ignored the edict and continued using amalgams. Many of them were expelled from the Society. Consequently, the American Society of Dental Surgeons lost its influence and by 1856 was disbanded.

In 1859 a new dental organization was formed—the National Dental Association, later renamed the American Dental Association (ADA). This organization favored the use of amalgam fillings and encouraged its members to use them. New dentists were taught that mercury fillings were safe. Although there were no studies to back it up, they were told that combining the mercury with other metals somehow locked it in place so that it posed no danger to the patient. With the backing of the ADA, filling teeth with mercury amalgams was accepted as a normal and presumably safe dental practice.

In the 1920s the amalgam controversy surfaced again. German chemist Alfred Stock, Ph.D., raised the alarm that mercury does in fact leach out of amalgams. Stock himself had mercury fillings, but when he suddenly began to experience neurological problems, he suspected it might be the fillings. He had the amalgams removed and almost immediately his symptoms went away. Convinced that mercury was the culprit, he began warning the medical and dental community. He demonstrated that mercury vapor was emitted from amalgam fillings and eventually published several scientific papers on the topic. His efforts, however, were met with severe opposition by the dental profession. He continued his campaign until the beginning of World War II. With the onset of the war, attention was drawn to other matters and the subject was soon forgotten.

Concern about mercury amalgams began to emerge again in the 1960s. Studies were being published that cast doubt on the safety of amalgam fillings. Researchers found that mercury vapor was constantly being emitted from dental fillings.[1-4]

The ADA, firm in its stance to protect the use of amalgams, insisted that mercury did not escape from fillings. Faced with increasing evidence to the contrary, they later revised their position. They admitted that some mercury vapor did escape, but only for the first week or so after the filling was placed in the tooth. Once the amalgam had fully hardened, the amount of vapor released was insignificant. Insignificant to whom? The ADA? Certainly not for the patient! Their proof was to point to a long history of safety. The problem with this argument is that amalgams rarely cause problems immediately. Symptoms occur gradually and often don't manifest themselves until years later. Who would suspect that

71

migraine headaches or multiple sclerosis (MS) that developed months or years after fillings were placed in the mouth were at the root of the problem?

According to the ADA reasoning, once an amalgam has hardened, it retains all of its mercury. This, however, is not true. The older the amalgams are, the less mercury they contain. Several studies have shown that older amalgams have lost as much as 80-90 percent of the mercury they once contained.[5]

The acids in saliva and foods constantly leach mercury out of the amalgams. Even chewing gum increases the release of mercury vapor. Tests show that after subjects have chewed gum for just 10 minutes, mercury vapor increases by over 15 fold.[6]

Heintze and colleagues discovered that oral bacteria convert mercury vapor into methylmercury, a highly toxic form of mercury and the same type that caused widespread sickness and death in Minamata, Japan from eating contaminated fish.[7]

The ADA claims that inhaling or ingesting small amounts of mercury vapor does not cause any harm. So how do they explain the many people who have had documented reactions to mercury fillings, or the many people who report recovery from chronic illness after having amalgams removed? The ADA claims that reactions occur only in a small number of people who are allergic or "sensitive" to mercury. What a ridiculous statement! Who is *not* sensitive to mercury? That's like saying you don't have to worry about eating arsenic or cyanide if you are not allergic to it. Mercury is a poison. Whether you are allergic to it or not, it is going to harm you.

Like oral bacteria, mercury can spread from the mouth to other parts of the body causing a wide range of symptoms and diseases. Evidence shows that mercury from amalgam fillings can contribute to a number of neurological problems, autoimmune diseases, and other health problems. Several European countries have restricted use of dental amalgam and ruled it shouldn't be used in pregnant women.

One of the conditions often associated with amalgams is MS. Multiple sclerosis is an autoimmune disease that slowly deteriorates nerve cells. Hal Huggins, D.D.S., author of *It's All in Your Head: The Link Between Mercury Amalgams and Illness*, recalls that after treating 50 cases of MS from a dental standpoint, someone told him he should write another book about the connection between MS and dental amalgams. Not certain at the time to what degree amalgams had in the overall incidence of MS, he responded, "When I have seen one thousand cases, I will write a book." A few years later he exceeded that number and decided it was time to write the book. It was published as *Solving the MS Mystery*.

According to Huggins, mercury toxicity may lead to a number of autoimmune diseases. Autoimmune disease is a condition in which a person's immune system attacks his or her own tissues. In addition to multiple sclerosis, other common autoimmune diseases include rheumatoid arthritis, lupus, diabetes (insulin-dependent), glomerulonephritis, Grave's disease, myasthenia gravis, Addison's disease, and Lou Gehrig's disease (ALS).

Your white blood cells are the workhorse of your immune system. Their job is to defend you from harmful substances. How do white blood cells tell the difference between your own cells and that of an intruder? Each cell in your body carries a special code, kind of like a license plate. This code is unique and belongs only to you. When white blood cells come into contact with another cell, they check its code to identify if it is "self" or "non-self." The code must match that of the white blood cell exactly to be recognized as "self." If it is identified as "self" nothing happens. If the code doesn't match, however, it is tagged as an intruder and promptly attacked.

Mercury has a special affinity for sulfur-containing amino acids. Amino acids are the basic building blocks for all proteins. Mercury can attach itself to amino acids on cell membranes. With mercury now a part of the cell, when a white blood cell comes by to read its code, the code reads self-plus mercury. Since this is not an exact match, the cell is identified as foreign and is attacked. In this way mercury can cause autoimmune disorders.

When mercury attaches itself to amino acids, it can cause all types of problems. Enzymes, which participate in thousands of chemical processes in the body, are made of amino acids. When mercury attaches itself to these enzymes, they become dysfunctional. This can disrupt all of the biological systems in the body to one degree or another, leading to any number of symptoms ranging from mental deterioration to chronic fatigue.

Mercury in the mouth is just as bad, if not worse than disease-causing bacteria or viruses. Removing amalgams from the mouth will stop the absorption of additional mercury into the body and reduce a heavy burden on the immune system. In many cases, patients report miraculous recoveries of chronic illness. My wife, Leslie, had suffered for many years with chronic migraine headaches. No amount of medication could relieve the pain. The migraines would persist for hours, totally incapacitating her. After she had her amalgams removed, the headaches disappeared almost immediately. She has been amalgam-free for over 10 years now and has not experienced a single migraine.

Leslie's story isn't unusual. Frank, a 61-year-old engineer, suffered from severe eczema, a stomach ulcer, repeated ear infections, chronic headaches, joint and back pains, tremors in his right arm and left leg, occasional chest pains, irregular heart beat, lack of concentration, and irritability. He had six teeth with amalgams and two nickel/porcelain bridges to compensate for several missing/damaged teeth. After reviewing his health history, his dentist suggested he remove the amalgams and exchange the nickel/porcelain bridges with ones made of gold and porcelain. Within days of the dental work he began feeling better. Over the next few weeks, he reported that all his symptoms had decreased remarkably, except his back pain and eczema, which increased in severity for a short period of time and then began to improve. After a few months, all of his symptoms ceased, including his chronic eczema and persistent earaches.

Not all patients who have amalgam fillings removed experience immediate results. When I had two amalgams removed from my mouth I didn't notice any change afterwards. But these amalgams had been in my mouth for about 35 years and, therefore, most all of the mercury had probably already leached out. Removing them didn't have a big impact on the toxic load in my body, but I still wanted them out because I felt that any amount of mercury wasn't good.

Sometimes the damage done is irreversible or takes an extended amount of time to heal. Our health is determined by many factors. Removing mercury fillings may be helpful, but does not guarantee immediate improvement in health. Mouth bacteria, diet, lifestyle, and environment can all influence health. The more issues you address, the greater your chance of improved health.

Dentists continue to place amalgam fillings into patient's mouths and may even strongly recommend them, telling you they are completely safe. Don't believe it. You should never, ever consider having amalgam fillings placed in your mouth. There are numerous new non-metallic composite materials available that are just as functional yet far safer. Unlike amalgams, they are white and match your teeth color so well you can't even tell you have a filling.

DENTAL MATERIALS

Numerous materials are temporarily or permanently placed in our mouths by dentists, some of which are relatively harmless, while others, like mercury amalgams, are potentially deadly. It is to your advantage to know which can do you harm and which are safest. There are hundreds of metal alloys that can be used in dentistry. Metals are used for fillings, crowns, partial dentures, orthodontics, and implants. Each manufacturer has their own formula for each item, so they can patent their products.

Some of the metals are more toxic than others. Anyone can be sensitive to any metal or alloy. Gold is generally the most benign of the metals. After testing nearly 4,000 patients, Dr. Hal Huggins says that he found that only nine percent have sensitivity to gold.[8] In comparison, 95 percent are sensitive to copper and 94 percent to zinc, both of which are components of amalgam fillings. So in addition to the mercury, the other metals in amalgam fillings can also cause problems.

If you do have metal placed in your mouth, you should make sure it is all of the same type. Two dissimilar metals can cause electrical energy to be generated inside your mouth. I recall reading years ago about a man who always heard music and talking in his head. No one else could hear it. On investigation, it was discovered that the metal in his mouth acted like a crude radio receiver, and he was receiving the broadcasts from a local station. Whether or not this story was factual I don't know, but it is not beyond belief. Metals in the mouth do produce electricity. Two or more dissimilar metals, combined with acids and electrolytes (ions in the saliva) produce an electrical charge just like a battery. Electricity is the flow of electrons. Electrons from one metal flow to the other. This causes the release of metallic ions into the mouth.

The release of potentially harmful metals like mercury, nickel, and copper is intensified.

Frequently, broken or root canalled teeth are built up or filled with amalgam to furnish a foundation for a crown to sit on. Placing gold over the amalgam (two dissimilar metals) stimulates mercury release. If you already have amalgam fillings, adding a gold filling will increase your mercury exposure. Likewise, adding a gold or nickel crown or a bridge containing nickel or any other metal dental work will do the same.

Nickel is a common dental metal used in crowns, bridges, and braces. So-called "chrome" crowns are really made of nickel-containing stainless steel. Like mercury, nickel is a toxic heavy metal, yet not as toxic as mercury. Nickel is immediately fatal at concentrations of 30 parts per million (ppm) or greater. The maximum allowable contaminant level set by the Environmental Protection Agency (EPA) for nickel in drinking water is 0.1 ppm. To put this number in perspective, the EPA's limit for arsenic is 0.01 ppm and for cyanide is 0.2 ppm. In other words, the EPA considers nickel to be one-tenth as toxic as arsenic but twice as toxic as cyanide.

If nickel is so toxic, why is it put in the mouth? Just like mercury, the ADA considers it to have lost it toxic properties when combined with other metals. What they don't consider is the fact that acids and electricity eat away at the metal, forming a corrosion soup that you swallow with your saliva.

Gold is a better choice in most cases for crowns and bridges. Composite materials are better for fillings than metals. Composites are made of a resin-based matrix with an inorganic filler, such as silica. There are many different types of composite materials.

If you need a filling, do not allow the dentist to put in amalgam. If he tries to talk you into it, go to another dentist. The best filling material is either gold or a composite, preferably the latter. However, you can't use just any composite material the dentist has on hand. You may be allergic or chemically sensitive to some of the composite materials, and you don't want to put something permanently into your mouth that you will have a bad reaction to. Therefore, you need to get a *compatibility test* done before getting the filling. The dentist will do this or refer you to someone who can. If your dentist says you don't need the test, he doesn't know what he is doing or doesn't care about your health. Find another dentist. During the compatibility test, you will have some blood drawn. With the blood, each composite material will be tested. You will then be given a list of those materials to which you had a positive reaction or a negative reaction. You should give this report to your dentist and he will select a compatible composite for you.

If you want existing amalgam fillings removed, you need to find a dentist who has been trained to do it properly. Most dentists are not. They can pull out the amalgam, but they will not do it properly? Removing mercury amalgam is dangerous. As the old filling is removed, mercury vapor and dust fills the air and your mouth! If the dentist does not take the necessary precautions, you can absorb huge amounts of mercury which can cause you more problems than if you had left the filling in place. You want to find a holistic or biological dentist who has been trained to remove amalgams properly. See the end of this chapter for guidance in finding a dentist who practices biological dentistry.

FLUORIDE

Fluorine is an element that in its purest form is a gas. When combined with other elements, it forms into a compound known as fluoride. Your dentist often uses fluoride when he works on your teeth. Your toothpaste likely contains fluoride, as do some mouthwashes. Fluoride is added to our drinking water. It is also the active ingredient in rat poison and cockroach powder.

Yes, fluoride is a poison. Fluoride is more poisonous than lead, and just less poisonous than arsenic.[9] For this reason, the Food and Drug Administration (FDA) mandates that a warning be placed on all fluoride-containing toothpaste. The warning states "Keep out of reach of children under 6 years of age" and if more than a pea sized amount of toothpaste is swallowed to "get medical help or contact a Poison Control Center right away." Why would anyone want to put something into his or her mouth that is so poisonous that swallowing just a pea-sized amount is dangerous enough to seek immediate medical attention?

Most people use much more than a pea-sized dab of toothpaste to brush their teeth. If fluoride is supposed to be absorbed into the teeth while we're brushing, won't it also be absorbed by the mucous membranes in the mouth, which are much more absorbent than teeth? Wouldn't that be just as bad as swallowing it?

We are warned that fluoride is dangerous and not to swallow it, yet when it is added to our drinking water we are led to believe that it suddenly loses its toxicity. Would you purposely drink water that has lead or arsenic added to it?

Fluoride is deliberately added to two-thirds of the US public water supplies, theoretically to reduce tooth decay. Outside the US, fluoridation has spread to Canada, the UK, Australia, New Zealand and a few other countries. The source of most of the fluoride that is added to municipal water supplies comes as a byproduct in the manufacture of aluminum, cement, steel, and phosphate fertilizers. Ordinarily, fluoride is treated as toxic waste and disposing of it is costly. In the 1930s researchers working for Alcoa Aluminum first suggested that 1 part per million (ppm) fluoride added to drinking water could reduce the incidence of dental cavities. This is interesting, because Alcoa produces tons of fluoride in the manufacture of aluminum. Finding a market for the fluoride would save them millions of dollars.

In Alcoa's eyes, the more fluoride that could be sold, the better. The 1 ppm figure was the highest level that could be added to drinking water without causing fluorosis—white spotted, yellow, brown and/or pitted teeth in more than about 10 percent of users.

Lobbying by Alcoa and its friends in government led to the fluoridation of public drinking water. In 1945 Newburgh, New York and Grand Rapids, Michigan became the first cities to test fluoridation. Consequently, fluoride became the first drug in history to be tested on the general population with no previous research to prove its safety.

The enamel in our teeth is composed predominately of calcium carbonate. When teeth are exposed to fluorine, it is absorbed directly into the enamel and becomes a part of it, forming calcium fluoride. "You have been led to believe that fluorine makes teeth harder," says Dr. George Meinig. "The fact is, it actually makes teeth softer. Any dentist who has treated numbers of people who have grown up in areas where the natural water supply is high in fluorine will testify that not only do these people's teeth develop fluorosis, an ugly brownish-grey stain throughout their enamel, but when these teeth are drilled they are obviously much softer than the teeth of most of the population. The

American Dental Association admits that when fluorine is added to the water supply at the recommended dose of one part per million, 10 percent of those using it have some degree of fluorosis. The reason teeth become softer is because calcium fluoride is not nearly so hard a structure as calcium carbonate. You would think teeth treated with fluorine would decay much more readily since they are soft. Calcium fluoride, however, is less soluble to attacks by acids then calcium carbonate, so acids created by the bacteria in the plaque are not so successful in etching the enamel, and the amount of decay is reduced. There is a feeling fluorine-treated teeth give protection against caries for a lifetime. Many studies have shown this protection disappears toward the end of the teenage years."

With the approval of such respectable organizations as the American Dental Association, Canadian Dental Association, the US Public Health Service, and Alcoa, you would think that there must be mountains of evidence that prove that fluoridation is safe and effective, right? Think again. If you want to stop a fluoridation advocate in his tracks, simply ask him to cite legitimate studies that prove fluoridation prevents tooth decay and is harmless at current rates of usage. The only evidence they can come up with are the original studies produced by Alcoa and their friends. More recent studies show that the effects on cavity prevention have been minimal. Good oral hygiene is just as effective and doesn't have all the detrimental effects associated with fluoride.

Fluoride is cumulative and toxic to all forms of life even at extremely low dosages. Double-blind studies prove adverse health effects at a 1 ppm level in water. Several recent studies suggest that fluoride consumption raises the risk of disorders affecting teeth, bones, the brain, and the thyroid gland.[10]

Even at current levels, about 5-10 percent of children develop the discoloration, pitting, and weakening of teeth characteristic of fluorosis. Dental fluorosis is more than a cosmetic problem. It is associated with increased tooth decay. So in some children fluoride in drinking water *increases* tooth decay. When you combine the fluoride in water with the exposure from other sources such as toothpaste, beverages, and medications, fluorosis rates can increase.

Drinking fluorinated water not only affects the teeth, but all the bones in the body. Since fluoride replaces carbonate in teeth, which causes them to become more brittle and weaker, it is reasonable to assume it does the same thing to bones. Population studies and tests on lab animals confirm this assumption.[11] Fluoride increases the risk of bone fracture, especially in vulnerable people, such as the elderly.[12]

"Fluoride causes bone disease—skeletal fluorosis—severe damage to the musculoskeletal and nervous systems resulting in muscle wasting, limited joint motion, spinal deformities, calcification of the ligaments, and neurological damage," says biochemist and bestselling author Lita Lee, Ph.D.[13] Despite calcium supplementation and increasing awareness and education about bone health, osteoporosis is on the rise. In the U.S. the hip fracture rate is now the highest on earth.

Fluoride is a common industrial pollutant that can kill both plants and animals. According to the U.S. Department of Agriculture, fluoride has caused more worldwide damage to domestic animals than any other air pollutant.[14] There has been more litigation on damage to agriculture by fluoride than all other pollutants combined.[15]

In the 1960s and 1970s, intentional dumping of massive quantities of fluoride into the air and water by Reynolds Metals Company and Alcoa caused severe fluoride poisoning on a Mohawk Indian reservation. Medical writer Joel Griffiths describes the result: "Cows crawled around the pasture on their bellies, inching along like giant snails. So crippled by bone disease, they could not stand up, this was the only way they could graze. Some died kneeling, after giving birth to stunted calves. Others kept on crawling until, no longer able to chew because their teeth had crumbled down to the nerves, they began to starve…The Mohawk children, too, showed signs of damage to bones and teeth."[16] The Mohawks filed a lawsuit against the companies but ended up settling out of court for barely enough to pay for the loss of their cows.

Weakened teeth and bones aren't the only problems with fluoride. The National Research Council (NRC) spent three years reviewing hundreds of studies on fluoride. They concluded that "fluoride can subtly alter endocrine function, especially in the thyroid—the gland that produces hormones regulating growth and metabolism." John Doull, professor emeritus of pharmacology and toxicology at the University of Kansas Medical Center, who chaired the NRC committee, said that the effects fluoride has on the thyroid "worry me."[17] They should, because fluoride can cause hypothyroidism.

"Fluoride causes cancer," says Dr. Lita Lee. "In 1981, Dean Burk (Chief Chemist at the National Cancer Institute) testified at congressional hearings that over 40,000 yearly cancer deaths are attributable to fluoridation. He said that *no chemical causes as much cancer, and faster, than fluorides.*" This information is well documented, verified and confirmed by epidemiological and animal studies.

Dr. Lee goes on to say, "The New Jersey Department of Health found that the risk of bone cancer was about three times as high in fluoridated areas as in nonfluoridated areas. This is because bone is a target for fluoride. The *Journal of Carcinogenesis* says that 'fluoride not only has the ability to transform normal cells into cancer cells but also to enhance the cancer-causing properties of other chemicals.'

"Fluoride causes genetic damage. An article in *Mutation Research* says that a study by Proctor and Gamble, makers of Crest toothpaste, did research showing that 1 ppm fluoride causes genetic damage. Results were not published.

"A National Institutes of Environmental Health Sciences publication, *Environmental and Molecular Mutagenesis*, also linked fluoride to genetic damage. 'Fluoride exposure in cultured human and rodent cells results in increased chromosome aberrations resulting in birth defects and the mutation of normal cells into cancer cells.'"

That's not all. Fluoride, even in minute doses, accumulates in and damages the brain and affects mental development in children. A series of epidemiological studies in China have associated high fluoride exposure with lower IQ.

Dr. Lee adds, "Fluoride poisons over 100 enzymes in your body. Fluoride disrupts collagen, the major connective tissue of the body, causing premature wrinkling and aging. Fluoride causes seizures in humans and animals."

It is ironic that fluoride is used to help reduce the occurrence of cavities, yet it has the potential to cause gum disease. Fluoride in toothpaste, mouthwashes, and water contribute to the formation of dental

Homemade Toothpaste (without fluoride)

Most commercial toothpaste contains fluoride, detergents, and other various chemicals. Brushing teeth doesn't require commercial toothpaste or any toothpaste at all for that matter. The abrasive action of the toothbrush alone is adequate for scouring off dental plaque. However, toothpaste that is properly formulated can aid in dental health. You can make your own toothpaste, without fluoride or harsh detergents, that is every bit as good, if not better, than commercial toothpaste. Use the following ingredients:

1 tablespoon baking soda
1 tablespoon vegetable glycerin
2-4 drops peppermint, wintergreen, or cinnamon oil
½ teaspoon xylitol (optional)

Baking soda is the primary component of this formula and works well for neutralizing acids and maintaining proper pH balance. It also acts as a mild abrasive. Glycerin provides a base to hold the baking soda and other ingredients together. It also tempers the salty-bitter taste of the baking soda. You can find glycerin at health food stores and pharmacies. Peppermint, wintergreen, and cinnamon oils help freshen the breath. Clove oil may be used as well. The advantage of the clove oil is that it is an effective disinfectant and can help reduce oral bacteria. Xylitol is optional. It helps sweeten the toothpaste, making it more palatable and also helps to kill germs.

Mix all the ingredients together; your toothpaste is now ready to use. This recipe makes enough toothpaste to last one person about 3 weeks. Since your homemade toothpaste does not contain gums and fillers, it will not look like commercial toothpaste. It will be more liquidly. Store the mixture in a small glass jar that has a sealable lid. The purpose of the lid is to keep out bugs and dust. Put the jar in your medicine cabinet. No refrigeration is required.

calculus or tarter—the hard mineral deposit on teeth that aggravates gum tissue, harbors bacteria, and stimulates chronic inflammation which can lead to gum disease.[18-19] What good is preventing cavities if you lose your teeth to gum disease? All it means is that the teeth you lose will be cavity free!

With all the risks associated with fluoride, what benefit does it offer? Are the benefits great enough to offset the numerous health risks now linked to its use? For adults the benefits are nil. In children who live in areas of the U.S. where the water is fluoridated, tooth decay rates are nearly identical to those who live in non-fluoridated areas.

Fluoridation and the use of fluoride toothpastes and related products are unnecessary and potentially harmful. Taking care of your teeth with regular brushing and daily oil pulling essentially eliminates any presumed need for fluoridated water or fluoridated toothpaste.

You can eliminate commercial products that contain fluoride, such as fluoride-containing toothpastes and mouth washes. If you live in an area that fluoridates its drinking water, you may want to consider other options. If you drink bottled water you may want to make sure it comes from a reliable source, as many brands are simply municipal water and may contain fluoride. Water distillers and reverse osmosis purifiers remove essentially all foreign particles, minerals, and toxins. However, they require several hours to produce one gallon of pure water, so you would have to prepare the water before you use it. Water filters are another option. You can have filtered water almost instantaneously, but not all water filters can remove fluoride, so check what the filter can do before making a purchase.

BIOLOGICAL DENTISTRY

If you are considering having existing amalgam fillings or root canalled teeth removed and are not quite certain about taking that step, I recommend that you study the issue further. Go to the bibliography at the back of this book for resources. Read some of the books by Huggins, Cutler, Ziff, and others. I also recommend going to the International

Center for Nutritional Research website www.icnr.com and reading the information they have on these issues.

Talk to your dentist. Most dentists, however, do not fully understand or appreciate the intimate connection between dental health and systemic health. The teeth are treated as an isolated segment of the body, as if they had no influence on overall health and well-being other than their role in digesting food. These dentists take the same view expressed by the ADA that mercury, root canals, and fluoride are harmless or even beneficial.

Dentists who understand the danger of mercury fillings and the issues regarding root canals and fluoridation will refuse to put amalgam fillings into patients' mouths. To them it is ethically irresponsible to put mercury in anyone's mouth. These dentists view your mouth as an integrated part of your entire body, and understand that the medical treatments performed on your mouth and teeth can have a huge impact on your overall health. This is the type of dentist you should talk to.

Dentists with this point of view have distinguished themselves from the rest by referring to their practice as biological dentistry. Other terms that are commonly used are mercury-free, environmental, and holistic dentistry. These dentists have continued their education and training to know how to safely and effectively remove amalgam fillings without causing the patient undue harm. If a dentist believes amalgams are harmless, he is going to be less cautious on their removal than a dentist who understands the danger. When amalgams are removed from the teeth, mercury vapor is released—you can't avoid it. The amount of mercury you absorb is determined by the procedures your dentist uses.

I recommend you seek out a dentist who has been trained in safe amalgam removal. Dr. Hal Huggins has perfected a method of amalgam extraction that is safe and brings about the quickest recovery from mercury-induced systemic disease. To find a dentist in your area contact Huggins Applied Healing by phone at 1 (866) 948-4638 (US and Canada) or visit www.hugginsappliedhealing.com.

Another resource is the Holistic Dental Association. The HDA is an international organization of mercury-free dentists. Their website offers a searchable database of members in the USA and worldwide.

Holistic Dental Association
PO Box 151444
San Diego, CA 92175 USA
(619) 923-3120
www.holisticdental.org

Not all holistically trained dentists are listed, only those who belong to this particular association. To find others you can do an Internet search. Search using the following terms:

biological dentistry
holistic dentistry
environmental dentistry
mercury-free dentistry

To search more specifically for someone in your area you can include the general location where you live, such as "biological dentistry Florida." If you live outside the USA, include in your search your country or use the biggest city nearest you, for example "biological dentistry London."

Chapter 5

The Miracle of Oil Pulling

A NEW THERAPY FROM TRADITIONAL MEDICINE

Oil pulling has its origins in Ayurvedic medicine of India. Ancient Ayurvedic medical texts (*Charaka Samhita* and *Sushrutha's Arthashastra*) dating back over 2,000 years describe it as "oil gargling." Long ago, Ayurvedic practitioners discovered that washing the mouth with vegetable oil not only cleanses the mouth but restores health to the body. The process is said to cure about 30 systemic diseases ranging from relatively minor problems like bad breath and headaches to more serious conditions such as asthma and diabetes.

The practice of rinsing the mouth with oil was so simplistic that it was often overlooked and did not receive the full attention it deserved. Dr. F. Karach, a physician who also practiced Ayurvedic medicine, brought oil gargling out of obscurity. Dr. Karach had perfected the Ayurvedic method of oil gargling and called his new version "oil pulling." Dr. Karach presented his findings on oil pulling at a conference held in the Ukraine, then a part of the USSR, to a group of oncologists (cancer specialists) and bacteriologists.

In this speech he outlined his method of oil pulling and described the remarkable power it had in curing a number of diseases. He claimed that through the simple method of oil pulling most illnesses could be totally cured and that it was unnecessary to use surgery and drugs, which often cause harmful side effects. The sucking or swishing of vegetable oil inside the mouth aids the body in healing itself. The process "pulls" toxins and germs out of the body and allows nature to take its course to bring about healing. He claimed that this technique heals migraine headaches, bronchitis, tooth pain, thrombosis, eczema, ulcers, cancer, intestinal diseases, heart and kidney diseases, encephalitis, paralysis, insomnia, women's diseases, chronic blood diseases, and diseases of the nerves, stomach, lungs, and liver.

He claimed that the oil therapy cured him of a chronic blood disease which he had suffered with for 15 years. In just three days it also cured his arthritis, which at times was so severe it was crippling. Dr. Karach said we live only half the length of time we could, suggesting that if we cleansed the body regularly though oil pulling we could extend our lifespan to 140 or 150 years.

Dr. Karach described his method. He recommended using refined sunflower oil, which is a common cooking oil used throughout India, but indicated that other oils could also be used. He believed that as the oil was being worked in the mouth, it draws toxins out of the bloodstream through the mucous membranes. After 15-20 minutes the oil is spit out and the mouth rinsed with water. As toxins are removed on a daily basis, it reduces stress on the immune system and allows the body to heal itself. Chronic and acute illnesses are cured.

Dr. Karach delivered his speech to a group of Western trained medical doctors steeped in the use of drugs, surgery, and radiation to treat illness. To them this strange new technique must have sounded preposterous. This method was so simple and his claims so remarkable that the audience must have questioned his sanity. If it wasn't for an article about Dr. Karach's talk that was published in a medical trade journal in Calcutta, India, in 1992, oil pulling as we know it might have remained in obscurity.

While taking a class on homeopathy, Tummala Koteswara Rao, a retired military officer residing in Bangalore, India, received a pamphlet on oil pulling based on the above article. In January of 1993, Mr. Rao and his wife began practicing oil pulling. "At the age of 63," says Rao, "I have cured myself of allergic sneezing and cold in the morning/night of over four decades, asthma, sleeplessness, palpitations, allergies due to food items, smells, and digestion problems of many years. My wife aged 56 was cured of three decades' old migraine headaches, four decades' old varicose veins and ulcers, arthritis, high blood pressure, and many other minor ailments. We suffered from the above diseases without hope, obtaining only temporary relief from different systems of medical treatment. Oil pulling cured our diseases without medicine after practicing it for just over a year."

Greatly impressed with the power of this simple technique, Rao was compelled to tell others about his success and promote the use of oil pulling as a means to restore good health. "I was obsessed with the idea that oil pulling should be brought to the notice of whoever was suffering with any disease," says Rao. He started distributing a pamphlet on oil pulling. Fortunately, a copy reached the editors of *Andhra Jyothi* a daily newspaper. Some of the editorial staff tried it, found it to be effective and published an article about this simple therapy. Rao volunteered to answer questions from readers. The response was so positive that the newspaper continued to publish weekly articles on the topic for three years. Other papers began publishing articles, creating an oil pulling health movement.

Over the course of 12 years Rao wrote numerous articles and gave over a thousand lectures. During this time he received more than 1,200 letters from people describing their experiences with oil pulling. He also met with a large number of people who personally related their experiences. "All of them," says Rao, "narrated how they suffered from one disease or another without cure from medical treatments, but were cured only by oil pulling."

Today Rao continues his campaign to educate people about the benefits of oil pulling. Although not a doctor or therapist, Rao believes the power behind oil pulling is based on the principles of Ayurvedic medicine and homeopathy and that oil pulling balances the energies within the body, bringing about cure.

While there may be an energy component involved, I believe there is a more physical mechanism involved: oral germs cause infections and disrupt body chemistry. Removing the germs relieves these conditions bringing about improved health.

WHERE'S THE PROOF?

One of the major criticisms of oil pulling, especially from the medical profession, is that there is little scientific proof that oil pulling works.

88

Doctors, on the whole, are very cautious about new or unproven therapies, especially when they challenge conventional practices. Funding institutions and pharmaceutical companies are not interested in verifying the effectiveness of natural therapies. Consequently, there has not been much published about oil pulling in standard scientific journals.

However, simply because there hasn't been much medical research on the topic, doesn't make it any less effective. The biggest worry doctors have about new treatments or therapies is the potential harm they might cause. Obviously, an untested drug or medical procedure could do great harm, so doctors are always cautious about anything new. They want it tested, retested, and tested again to prove its safety before recommending it to their patients. This precaution isn't necessary with oil pulling because it is totally harmless and has a proven safety record extending back at least 2,000 years. Nobody ever died or suffered any type of harm by swishing vegetable oil in their mouths. You are not even swallowing the oil, so you don't ingest anything. Oil pulling is one of the most nonintrusive, least harmful, and simplest forms of treatment in existence. Yet, it is also one of the most powerful and most effective.

Although there may not be a lot of medical research published on oil pulling, that does not mean there is no evidence for its effectiveness and safety. Actually, there is a good deal of evidence. We know that the mouth is a breeding ground for germs. We know that germs in the mouth can migrate to other parts of the body, cause infections, and alter body chemistry, leading the way to any number of infectious and

Oral Hygiene

Teeth represent only 10 percent of the surface of your mouth and bacteria live throughout the whole mouth. When you stop brushing, bacteria left behind resettle on your teeth and gums. Oil pulling reaches virtually 100 percent of the mouth, thereby affecting all bacteria, viruses, fungi, and protozoa in the mouth.

degenerative conditions. There are hundreds of published medical studies to prove this. We also know that oil pulling removes germs from the mouth, reducing the number that can enter into the body to cause harm. This is plainly evident to anyone who tries it. We know the human body has an amazing capacity to heal itself and will, if given the opportunity. Oil pulling provides this opportunity by reducing the toxic load on the body and unencumbering the immune system so it can work more efficiently. The fact is that thousands of people have experienced improvement. If it is harmless and works, why knock it? Instead, do it yourself, and gain the benefits.

Andhra Jyoti Survey

There have been a few published studies on the effectiveness of oil pulling. The first was a survey conducted by and published in *Andhra Jyoti* in 1996. *Andhra Jyoti* is the daily newspaper that ran Tummala Koteswara Rao's weekly column on oil pulling for several years. The editors asked readers who had tried oil pulling to participate. The purpose of the survey was to find out the effectiveness of the treatment and what types of diseases it cured.

Out of a total of 1,041 respondents, 927 (89%) reported being completely cured of one or more diseases. Only 114 (11%) people reported no significant improvement. The analysis indicated cures from the following conditions:

Aches and pains in the body, neck, and head .... 758 cases
Allergy and respiratory problems like asthma
    and bronchitis .... 191 cases
Skin problems such as abnormal pigmentation,
    itching, and eczema .... 171 cases
Digestive problems .... 155 cases
Constipation .... 110 cases
Arthritis and joint pain .... 91 cases
Diabetes .... 56 cases
Hemorrhoids .... 27 cases
Female hormonal problems .... 21 cases
Other diseases like cancer, polio, leprosy, polycystic
    kidney, neural fibroma, paralysis .... 72 cases

As you look at the responses, please keep in mind that those conditions that are most prevalent in the population are the ones that indicate the greatest number of cures. Those conditions that are less common, like diabetes and cancer, show fewer cures because there are fewer people who have these conditions. It is interesting that the terminology of the survey stated complete "cures," and not just "improvement."

Although the survey wasn't conducted under strict scientific parameters, it still provides strong evidence for the effectiveness of the therapy.

Pioneer Match Industries Study

In 2005 Pioneer Match Industries in Tamil Nadu, India conducted a study on oil pulling involving the female employees in their factory. Out of about 150 female workers who started the study, a total of 144 completed it. Oil pulling and its benefits were explained to the employees. They were given oil, without cost, and told to use it daily on an empty stomach. Oil pulling was usually done once each morning before breakfast.

After 25 days the women reported their results. They did not list specific ailments but rated the effectiveness of the treatment in relieving symptoms associated with any health problems or concerns they had. Each rated their results in one of four categories—very good, good, average, or no effect. The results were as follows:

Effect	Number of Workers	Percent
Very good	23	16
Good	58	40
Average	56	39
No effect	7	5

A total of 137 (93 percent) indicated some improvement and 81 workers (56 percent) indicated good or very good results. Only seven participants (5 percent) indicated no benefit. This study was limited to just 25 days. If the study had lasted longer it would have undoubtedly produced a higher positive effect. This study corresponds well with the

Andhra Jyoti Survey where there were 89 percent who indicated improvement and 11 percent with no noticeable improvement.

Participants indicated improvement in a variety of conditions just as respondents did in the Andhra Jyoti Survey. One woman had an exceptional response. She was one of the supervisors, age 35, with two children. She was diabetic and had been taking medications for the condition for the last two years. As she began oil pulling, her blood sugar levels began to improve. After 20 days she was able to reduce her medication by 50 percent and still keep her blood sugar within normal. Encouraged, she continued with the therapy when the study was completed. After 20 more days of oil pulling she discontinued all medication. Blood sugar levels remained normal, energy levels were higher, and her performance at work improved.

KLES Institute Study

The first study to appear in a scientific journal on the effects of oil pulling was published by the *Journal of Oral Health and Community Dentistry*.[1] Dr. H.V. Amith and colleagues at the Department of Preventive and Community Dentistry at the KLES Institute of Dental Sciences in Belgaum, India conducted this study.

Their objective was to assess the effect of oil pulling on plaque and gingivitis and to monitor its safety on the teeth and gums. This study is important because it provides a direct link between oil pulling and systemic disease. If oil pulling has any effect in reducing the number of microorganisms entering the body, it must first be able to reduce the amount of bacteria in the mouth and have a positive effect on common oral problems such as dental plaque and gum disease. If it doesn't, then oil pulling may be useless. If it does, however, we have direct evidence that oil pulling can affect systemic conditions caused by oral focal infections.

Ten subjects, physiotherapy students at the university, participated in the study. The age range was 19-21 years. This was a blind study in that the subjects were not told the purpose of the investigation in order to avoid any possible bias. All the subjects chosen had mild to moderate gingivitis and plaque accumulation, were free from systemic disease, and were not using any medications. They were instructed to continue their normal home oral hygiene practices, along with oil pulling. Oil pulling was performed once each morning for a period of 45 days. Plaque levels and the severity of gingivitis were assessed periodically during the study.

The subjects were instructed to take 10-15 ml (2-3 teaspoons) of refined sunflower oil using a spoon. They were to sip, suck and pull the oil through the teeth for 8-10 minutes before spitting it out.

At the end of the 45 days no adverse reactions to the teeth or soft tissues in the mouth were found, indicating that the procedure caused no physical harm. Most people would have assumed this, but the study gave confirmation. Plaque formation was significantly reduced, with most of the reduction coming during the later half of the study, indicating that the longer you do the treatment the better the results. Gingivitis was also significantly reduced in all subjects, decreasing by more than 50 percent. The researchers rated the changes as "highly" significant and stated that this study "proved" that oil pulling has dental benefits.

Mouthwashes have shown to reduce plaque by 20-26 percent and gingivitis by about 13 percent. Tooth brushing reduces plaque by 11-27 percent and gingivitis by 8-23 percent.[2] Oil pulling beats them both. Data from this study shows that oil pulling reduced plaque by 18-30 percent and gingivitis by an amazing 52-60 percent. The reduction in plaque using oil pulling is only slightly better than antiseptic mouthwashes and brushing, but reduction in gingivitis is two to seven times greater. So, oil pulling significantly out-performs brushing and mouthwash as a means of oral cleansing.

Reduction of Dental Plaque and Gingivitis with Various Treatments (%)		
Treatment	Dental Plaque	Gingivitis
Tooth Brushing	11-27	8-23
Antiseptic Mouthwash	20-26	13
Oil Pulling	18-30	52-60

While oil pulling can significantly reduce plaque and gingivitis, the authors caution it shouldn't be used in place of tooth brushing, but can be an effective supplemental aid in a daily oral hygiene regimen.

Other Published Studies

As might be expected, the greatest amount of research activity on oil pulling is occurring in India, where oil pulling has become exceptionally popular. Other studies from research intuitions in India confirm the findings of the KLES Institute Study.

In order to reduce plaque and gingivitis, the bacteria that cause these conditions must be reduced. That was the focus of the following studies. Researchers at Meenakshi Ammal Dental College in Chennai, India set out to determine the effect of oil pulling on *Streptococcus mutans* (S. mutans), the bacteria primarily responsible for dental plaque and cavities. Ten subjects were instructed to oil pull for 10 minutes every morning before brushing. S. mutans populations were measured in dental plaque and saliva after 24 hours, 48 hours, 1 week, and 2 weeks.

The researchers found that oil pulling significantly affected S. mutans populations. Researchers stated, "In this study there was a definitive reduction in the S. mutans count in plaque and saliva after oil pulling therapy" and indicated that oil pulling would be a useful tool in maintaining oral hygiene.[3]

The researchers admitted that they didn't know exactly how oil pulling worked, but suggested that the viscosity of the oil could possibly inhibit bacterial adhesion and plaque formation or that the emulsified mixture of oil and saliva and acted like a detergent and removed bacteria much like soap and water does when washing the hands.

A similar study was conducted by researchers at V.H.N.S.N. College in Virudhunagar, India. In this study the effect of oil pulling on the reduction of S. mutans and L. acidophilus was determined. Ten subjects with active dental cavities were selected. Bacterial populations were measured before and after oil pulling. After forty days of oil pulling once daily, total bacteria count was reduced up to 33 percent in the participants.

The researchers concluded that oil pulling was "effective in reducing bacterial growth and adhesion."[4] They, too, recommended oil pulling as a useful means for maintaining oral hygiene.

Another study conducted at Meenakshi Ammal Dental College evaluated the affects of oil pulling on S. mutans populations in dental plaque and saliva of 20 teenage boys.[5] Like the previous studies, the researchers concluded that "there was a definitive reduction in the S. mutans count in plaque and saliva after oil pulling therapy." Although they did not know exactly how oil pulling accomplished this, they theorize that the oil probably inhibits bacterial adhesion and plaque coaggregation. Another possible mechanism they suggested was saponification or the "soap-making" process that occurs as a result of alkali hydrolysis of fat. When the oil is acted upon by salivary alkalis like bicarbonate, the soap producing process is initiated. Soaps are good cleansing agents because they are active emulsifiers. Emulsification is the process by which insoluble fats like vegetable oil can be broken down into minute droplets and dispersed in water. Emulsification greatly enhances the surface area of the oil, thereby increasing its cleansing action.

As the popularity of oil pulling continues, more studies are bound to appear in medical and dental journals around the world. These studies will undoubtedly provide additional evidence of the effectiveness of oil pulling as a means of preventing and treating oral and systemic infections.

SUCCESS STORIES

Perhaps the most convincing and motivating evidence for the effectiveness of oil pulling are the personal testimonies of hundreds of people who have done it. A therapy isn't any good if it can't produce results; oil pulling produces results. The quickest and most obvious results are improvements in oral health—cleaner teeth, fresher breath, healthy pink gums, and less bleeding. Oral infections are reduced or eliminated followed by an improvement in systemic conditions. The following testimonies illustrate some of the many miracles of oil pulling (OP).*

*Testimonials from Soreena, Peggy, Paige, Diane, Paul, Jenny, Mark, Dan, Valerie, Sylvia, Maya, A.R., Arlene, Angel, Taylor, Alice, Lara, Willia, and Annette on pages 96-106 herein originally appeared on www.earthclinic.com's oil pulling section.

Oral Health

I decided to try oil pulling last Saturday as opposed to an antibiotic. I have an infection in my jawbone from a bad crown placed a year ago. I looked like a chipmunk and was in a lot of pain. I pulled twice Saturday, three times Sunday and three times a day since. By Monday morning my jaw was normal and I could chew on that side for the first time in months. I still have a lump in the bone but no more pain. I don't know if it does everything else it claims, but I know it took my infection away.

Theresa

I've noticed my teeth are much whiter and my tongue is the healthiest pink I have ever seen it to be. Oh! I seem to be passing food better. Not to be graphic, but have been having normal eliminations in the morning right after OP and also in the evening right before going to bed. I am only oil pulling in the mornings, first thing for 20 minutes, on an empty stomach.

C. W.

I had immediate relief from a tooth injury from a bad dentist. I can't really explain how it works, but I also sleep better, too. I used extra virgin olive oil first and then sesame seed oil. When I first did it, the tooth pain stopped. I had a terrible taste of metal in my mouth which is one of the reasons I really knew this was pulling toxins out. I also felt very weak and run down for the first two days and then very energetic!

Sorenna

I have been doing oil pulling for about one month and using cold pressed walnut oil. I went into the dentist for my semi-annual cleaning and exam. Both the hygienist and the dentist commented on how healthy my gums have become. My dentist said "whatever you're doing, it's working." In the past I have had a problem with bleeding gums—that is *gone*.

Peggy

For about two years I was unable to chew on the right side of my mouth because of tooth pain and extreme sensitivity to hot, sweet, cold, etc. I strongly suspect I am in need of another root canal. Starting with the second day of oil pulling I found the entire right side of my mouth was no longer sensitive. Beginning with the third day, I was able to chew on the right side of my mouth, albeit gingerly. Now, three weeks later I chew on the right side of my mouth equally with the left side— no pain, no sensitivity. And I've noticed my teeth feel more secure and they no longer feel loose.

Paige

I have been oil pulling two times a day for about a month now and notice a vast improvement in my gums. I have had two root canals and at my last dental visit, they wanted to do a third root canal to correct the previous two. Needless to say, I had severe gum pain and an abscess that caused me excruciating pain. My jaw would swell up to the size of a chipmunk's. I was in constant pain. I started oil pulling with sunflower oil and noticed that my pain had decreased intensity by day three. Within seven days, I had no pain and my abscess was completely gone. I ran out of sunflower oil and am now using extra virgin coconut oil. My gums are a healthy pink—they are no longer receding. I had a loosened tooth that really needed to be pulled but the gums have tightened around the tooth and it is no longer loose. My skin feels softer and I'm no longer plagued with earaches.

Diane

Infections

I tried oil pulling for the first time this morning and it had an incredible effect on my thrush (oral candida). Not only that, but my gums have already almost completely stopped bleeding. I've been on medicine after medicine for thrush but each one makes it worse and the doctors were stumped. One session of oil pulling (I only did it for 5 minutes to start off) has gotten rid of most of my thrush except the thick parts in the back of my tongue. This is truly amazing.

Paul

About 8 months ago, my wisdom teeth were giving me so much pain I could barely speak, much less eat. The dentist would tell me to go to a surgeon to get them removed and the surgeon would tell me to see my dentist because they weren't out enough to be removed! After about 2 weeks of this non-sense, a friend told me to try oil pulling. After the first 4 days, I started seeing results! My teeth weren't hurting so much and they felt cleaner. I haven't visited a dentist since then, nor any other doctor. I haven't even gotten a cold this year!! I used to get a cold or fever or sinus infections (you name it) every few months with the change in the weather, but not this year! I had a sore throat 2 weeks ago but that lasted 2 days and I was better already! My face looks brighter and I feel more energized as well. I would recommend this to anybody, whether you have problems or not. It's absolutely amazing! I feel healthier now than I did 5 years ago!

Jenny

Since early childhood I have had the herpes simplex virus in my body and suffered from frequent cold and canker sores. Now, by the time I feel one on my tongue it is gone in the morning. The other day the smallest, single-blister cold sore I ever had, which was all but invisible, appeared in the corner of my mouth. It went through its stages and was absolutely gone in three days, flat. Without treatment the blisters multiply and the healing process normally takes around two weeks.

Paige

Allergies and Asthma

I have missed weeks from work due to allergies in the last year…I started oil pulling and I could really see the toxins leaving my body through mucous, etc. After two weeks my allergies have been cured and I feel great.

Mark

I have been suffering from allergy and asthma from the age of 11 years when I had my first menses…It was very severe. This was lasting for about 3-4 days every month. I had tried all types of treatment for 45 years to get rid of this but without any success. I was spending my life with medicines but without cure…Two months after practicing (OP) my problems of health became a little more severe and I took them as healing reactions and consoled myself with the hope that I am going to be cured totally after the reactions. These reactions lasted for about two months. Now after nine months of OP I have become wonderfully healthy. Asthma has gone, no pains in the joints or body, no spots or discoloration of the skin, instead the skin has acquired a new shine, digestion has improved and I can eat anything without the fear of allergy.

V. L.

About two weeks ago I was taking my inhaler about twice a day. Then I started oil pulling. You can draw your own conclusions. But all I can say is that the very next day I stopped having to use my inhaler. I didn't experience an immediate throwing-up of mucus. But what I did experience is a gradual coughing-up of mucus all throughout the day. Another thing that I've experienced at least twice is what happens if my chest becomes tight. Usually when my chest tightens it'll stay that way and gradually gets worse until I take my inhaler. What I'm seeing is that when my chest tightens, I'll go through maybe a three hour period where I'll slowly begin to cough-up mucus until my chest is clear again. I have NEVER experienced my chest clearing-up all by itself after it has tightened. I've ALWAYS had to take medicine in order to get relief. During that time, my nose was stuffed a lot of the time. Since I've been OP-ing, it hasn't been. I can only conclude that it must be due to the oil pulling.

Dan

Sinuses

I was not able to sleep under a fan or in the open as my nose used to block. Cold-water bath was another curse. After practicing OP, I am able to sleep right under the fan with full speed with no discomfort. The occasional asthmatic or esoinophilia attacks vanished. Pain which I've had on my left knee and right ankle for three to four years is no longer there. A small five-year-old eruption on my skull vanished and twenty-year-old case of hemorrhoids has miraculously vanished.

T. R.

I've been oil pulling for 12 days and taking coconut oil for 10. I'm thrilled with the results. On the second day of OP my sinuses started to drain (didn't know they were congested) and two days later my lungs started to expel mucous. Also found that I was sleeping much better and had more energy. Of course, the mouth and teeth felt great. I am taking coconut oil about 3 times a day. It is all absolutely astounding.

Valerie

I started OP two weeks ago. The results are amazing. My sinus problems have cleared up after much mucus building and spitting the first few days. Sinus meds are now a thing of the past. My teeth are brighter and my gums no longer bleed when I brush my teeth.

Sylvia

The audible wheezing noises while breathing whenever I would lie down have stopped. I seem to be sleeping better too…My lungs no longer feel congested and I have no coughing fits anymore while trying to expel the congestion out of my lungs. I had been a heavy smoker for twenty-some years before quitting 18 years ago and this is probably the genesis of my lung problems.

Paige

Digestion

I am 82 years old. I have been suffering from constipation and hemorrhoids for the last four decades. I consulted many doctors, used many medicines but with only temporary relief. Within two weeks of practicing OP, I started getting relief. There was no pain during motion. Inflammation and hemorrhoids decreased. I started having free and clear evacuations. I am sleeping peacefully and happily at night. Indigestion, lack of appetite has gone. Decade's old pain has gone just by doing OP.

N.R.

I had recently suffered from left ventricular failure. After 15 days of starting OP, I could find the change in my condition as evidenced by the echocardiogram. I was suffering from acid peptic disease (duodenal ulcer) for the past 30 years, and OP has miraculously given relief and I have stopped using antacids. I had benign hypertrophy of the prostate for some years, and after OP nocturnal frequency of urine is much reduced. Some minor ailments like stomatitis (inflammation of the mucus membrane of the mouth), glossitis (inflammation of the tongue), itching of skin on the chest and neck, and discoloration of the skin have also gone. After OP, I saw that my palms appeared bright and full-blooded. So I went to the laboratory and got my HB tested. I was surprised to see that the hemoglobin content of my blood has risen from 11 to 12.4

grams within a period of two months.

Dr. N. Ranga Rao (surgeon)

Diabetes/Blood Sugar

I weigh 90 kilos (180 pounds), height 4'11" with weak twisted foot. By walking, the foot used to become septic and pus used to ooze. By OP and walking daily, I became strong and was able to walk up the steps without difficulty. OP reduced blood sugar gradually and diabetes cured. The skin became clear and shining and the spots on the body disappeared. The body became strong, teeth firm; gums healthy and the hair turned black and stopped becoming white or gray.

A.U.

At the advanced age of 74, it is unjust to expect miraculous results from any kind of therapy. Yet, I must say that what I have experienced through OP therapy is almost a miracle and quite unbelievable. Diabetes has been troubling me for the past 13 years. Now my blood sugar level is normal, though I do not take any medicine. I have discontinued all medication including vitamins, enzymes, etc.

S.B.

Joint Pain/Arthritis

I have been suffering from arthritis in the knees for the last 10 years and pain in the lower back for the last two decades. I have tried several allopathic medicines and got temporary relief. I started doing OP…and observed miraculous changes happening. Within five days my arthritis in the knees and lower back pain are completely cured. It is just unbelievable.

S.J.G.

I tried it just yesterday and was shocked at how fast results can be observed! I'm suffering from a knee injury due to my active lifestyle and since I'm not exactly young, I don't recover too easily. I've been having a bad knee for weeks now. But when I did my first oil pulling yesterday, I got immediate results! My knee felt so light and I was able to do squats with no problems! I'm really a skeptic so I was finding ways to credit the improved knee flexibility to other health practices of mine. But when my mom tried it later that night (she suffers for acute arthritis), she too said her joints felt remarkably better.

Maya

I am 71 years old, neck hurt since I was 12 yeas old. I haven't slept with a pillow for 31 years. The first week (after starting OP) my neck stopped hurting, and I slept with a pillow, second week I gave up my heating pad that I used for 40 years.

A.R.

I have been pulling for about 2 months now, the best thing that I noticed is the knee pain in both knees is completely gone. My feet don't hurt when I first get up to walk after sitting. I have recommended this to one of my employees that was having extreme pain in his legs. He reported to feel much better after just a few days. I will continue this from now on. I pull oil while taking my shower and doing my morning routine. My skin is much clearer.

Debbie

I had back pain for the past ten years and have been taking treatment for the same with several doctors and traction was also given for sufficiently long time without any improvement. I never used to go to bed without a medicine like Brufen, Voveran, and others daily...I started practicing OP with sunflower refined oil and started finding improvement within fifteen days and I was much relieved of the pain within three months. Now it is six months since I have been doing it and 90 percent of the pain is relieved. Now along with the back pain, the pain in my neck and armpits is also gone. I am not taking any medicine for the back pain.

Dr. V. Prabhakar

Skin

I OP with virgin coconut oil every morning. Makes my teeth white, my gums firm, makes the skin on my face soft, reduced acne and most strangely removed a mark/blemish on my arm that I've had there since I was a kid, 20 years there and gone within three weeks. I'm a firm believer.

S.H.

Since oil pulling I have had no breakouts on my face! It's amazing! My face is really looking good. That is enough to keep me at it. I've also gotten compliments that my teeth are whiter too! Love it!

J.L.

I am 79 years retied teacher...I wanted to be healthy by doing OP and have been practicing once daily...I've had eczema for the last 30 years on my left foot. It has been there in spite of various treatments. Similarly, had eczema on my right index finger for the last 10 years. I have had lower back pain for quite a few years. It is called spondylitis. I have been OP for the last year and 8 months. Lower back pain has completely gone. Eczema on the right index finger is also cured and skin is normal. The eczema on the left foot is becoming normal with a little itching sometimes. I am sure it will also go, but the cure is simply surprising.

C.V.R.

I started oil pulling three months ago to see what it could do. Immediately I noticed much whiter teeth. Within the week, my tongue and gums were pinker and healthier looking. The pale white coating that had been on my tongue for years was decreasing the more I oil pulled. My joints lost their stiffness, to the degree that I no longer take MSM Glucosamine or need to use my foot massager to relieve their stiffness. I was starting to walk like an old lady, and this was great to be free of that!

My skin became softer and smoother all over. For decades I had a skin condition—keratosis pilaris—little bumps all over my upper arms and cheeks. This had decreased by 99 percent and I can wear sleeveless tops again without embarrassment.

I took a trip to visit my sister for 3 weeks, and cut back my oil pulling to 10 minutes each morning so we could start chatting as soon as we got up. The bumps started to come back. I resumed the 20 minute regimen, and they again diminished. For me, this was conclusive evidence that it was the oil pulling responsible for the clearer skin.

K.P.

Sleep, Energy, and Weight Loss

I'm on my fourth day of oil pulling. I have noticed that my mouth is the cleanest it has ever been and man, are they getting white! I am sleeping better and having energy in the morning because of it.

H.D.

I have noticed increased metabolism, teeth tightening, and weight loss of 12 pounds since starting the oil pulling. I have so much more energy, teeth seem to be whitening. A clearer mind. The weight loss has been the best for me.

Arlene

I tried the sesame and then the sunflower oils, and then someone mentioned virgin coconut oil, well I find this to be my favorite. I am 5 foot 2 inches and generally have a stable weight of 51 kg (100 pounds), but over the last few months I've lost about 5 kg (10 pounds).

Peggy

I've been doing this for less than a week, once before breakfast. This morning when I weighed myself, I saw that in the week I have lost 1.5 kg (3 pounds). I have a lot of excess weight, so that is really welcome.

Vera

I was suffering from a sinus infection for 3 months and taking Dayquil everyday just to get through the day. After one time of OP my sinus drained immediately, I didn't have to wait. I stopped the meds that day, continued to OP, mucus pulled out everyday. I am amazed. Also my teeth, gums, and tongue are cleaner than ever. A couple of things I didn't expect: my energy has skyrocketed, even in the morning (it has been at least 20 years since I've had energy like this without caffeine). Also I don't crave caffeine, sugar, or salt. I sleep restful and don't need as much sleep. My skin is as soft as a baby. I was hooked on monster energy drinks, I drank at least 3 a day, but none since OP.

Angel

Hormones

I normally get acne blemishes on my chin and cheek area during my periods because of the hormone changes. But for these past two months I've been oil pulling, I am not breaking out whatsoever!
N.K.

I thought oil pulling sounded weird at first, but then a PhD friend of mine emailed me and told me she started oil pulling, and that's about the time I decided I should try it too. I started oil pulling and have no intentions of ever stopping it. It has helped my sleep, moods, reduced my anxiety, improved my brain function, and more.
Ellen

I have been doing oil pulling for one month. I read that it helps hormonal problems, but I didn't think it would eradicate my cramps. But after pulling for 1 month, my menstrual cramps and other PMS associated problems are almost nonexistent. For the first time in years I was able to spend the first day of my course like any other normal day, not bent over in agonizing pain. And my skin has cleared up as well. My sister started OP and after a week she had the same outcome! No cramps.
Taylor

I've been oil pulling for a little over two months now. Here are some of the things OP has helped me with: PMS, my cramps are almost completely gone now! I used to live on ibuprofen but I didn't even take it this time. Bloating, non-existent. Gas, nearly gone! Extremely tired in the mornings, gone. Oil pulling is one of the most amazing things. I wish everyone could learn about it!
Alice

I suffered from severe irregular periods that were very dark. I would get my period like once every two or three months. My hormones were completely off. I was out of balance. After my first month of oil pulling my periods came about 6 weeks apart. That was like unheard of for me for years. The next month my cycle came exactly 28 days after. And I have since had regular cycles for the past four months. The cycles are regular and bright, not dark or clotty anymore.

Lara

Headaches

For years I have suffered from migraine headaches. I have had migraines that hung on for days. Nothing would provide lasting relief. When a migraine finally did go away, his brother from Hell was sure to arrive!!! Well, oil pulling just knocked out my migraine in 10 minutes flat!!!

E.A.

Fibromyalgia

I tried it and it worked wonders for my fibromyalgia pain. I used the recommended amount 2 tbsp; swished it around in my mouth for 15 minutes, spit it out, brushed my teeth and drank two glasses of water. I have TMJ—I did not think I would be able to do this for 15 minutes due to jaw pain but after 2 ½ minutes my jaw pain left. The stiffness, pain and soreness in my body was gone before the 15 minutes was up. I have been suffering from fibromyalgia since 1991 and this is the only thing I have tried that gave me immediate relief.

Willia

Multiple Conditions

I have been oil pulling for 2 months 1 to 2 times daily. I have noticed several benefits: Immediately my gums stopped bleeding when flossed. My teeth felt more firmly seated in my gums, and they are whiter. After a month, my skin on my neck and chest improved in smoothness and elasticity (chicken bumps gone). I have a few moles on my body that are shrinking! My elbows are so smooth. Improved morning breath odor. Cravings for caffeine diminished. Improved joint mobility. I had a fingernail that I had mashed in a car door 25 years ago that never fully grew back and it is almost fully reattached! Dandruff is gone after 2 months of regular OP.

Annette

Chapter 6

Oil Pulling Basic Training

Teeth are meant to last a lifetime and they will if they are taken care of properly. Since our earliest years, we have been taught about the importance of oral hygiene and instructed to brush our teeth and floss daily. Most of us, however, never imagined how crucial oral hygiene is to the health of our entire body. Despite brushing, flossing, and regular visits to the dentist, our dental health on the whole is poor. Yes, we can have a bright smile, with straight, white teeth, but appearances can be deceiving. With the wonders of modern dentistry, our mouths can look healthy, but behind those pearly whites may lurk a toxic waste dump.

Gum disease and tooth decay are far more prevalent than most of us realize. U.S. statistics reveal that by the age of 17, about 60 percent have early signs of gum disease, and by the age of 50, up to 80 percent of the population is affected, with half suffering the severest form. Worldwide about 90 percent are affected. Dental health in most people is so poor that by age 65, one out of every three people have lost *all* of their teeth. When you are 65, how many teeth will you have remaining in your mouth? Regardless of how much care you take or how good your teeth may look, chances are right now you have some level of gum disease or tooth decay.

You don't need to have a root canal or an abscessed tooth to spread infection to other parts of your body. Bacteria in the mouth can spread as a result of just about any type of dental procedure, including brushing your teeth.[1] When gums are inflamed, they bleed easily, bristles from even the softest toothbrush can tear tiny blood vessels in the gums, leaving the door wide open for bacteria to enter into your bloodstream.

Traditional methods of oral hygiene have proven inadequate, as evidenced by the high incidence of gum disease (90 percent) and the ever-increasing incidence of oral-related systemic diseases (heart disease, arthritis, asthma, etc.). Oil pulling offers an excellent way to reduce microbial populations and improve oral and systemic health.

OIL PULLING STEP-BY-STEP

Oil pulling is very simple. All you do is take a spoonful of vegetable oil and swish it in your mouth. I recommend that you use liquefied coconut oil. Use 2-3 teaspoons of oil (1 teaspoon = 5 ml). The amount you use depends on what feels comfortable to you. Three teaspoons (1 tablespoon) is too much for many people; two teaspoons is about right. You don't want to take too much because you need to leave room for the secretion of saliva.

Keeping your lips closed, work the oil in your mouth; suck, push, and pull the oil through your teeth and over every surface of your mouth. Be relaxed, but keep the oil and saliva working constantly in your mouth for a total of 15-20 minutes. This may sound like a long time, but if you do other things at the same time, it doesn't seem so long. It seems that the longer you pull, the more effective it is. Some people have observed that if they pull for a full 20 minutes certain health problems go away, but if they reduce the time to less than 10 minutes, their problems may return.

Do not gargle the oil! Gargling may cause you to swallow some of the oil and trigger a gag reflex, causing you to spit the whole mouthful out. It may even cause you to vomit.

Do not swallow the oil. It is full of bacteria and toxins. You don't want that in your stomach. If you inadvertently swallow a portion while you are pulling, don't worry—it won't kill you—but avoid it if possible. As you swish the oil, your mouth secretes saliva; the saliva mixes with and almost emulsifies the oil, turning the mixture a milky white color. If the oil is not milky white, you didn't "work" it enough in your mouth.

Generally, it takes only a few minutes of vigorous pulling for the oil to turn color.

Sometimes mucous may form in the back of your throat as you are pulling. You don't want to choke. If needed, spit out the oil and clear your throat of the mucous. Get another mouthful of oil and continue. You don't need to start all over; go until you have done a total of about 20 minutes.

As saliva fills your mouth, you may run out of room before you are ready to stop. You can spit the whole thing out and take another spoonful, or you can simply spit out a portion and keep pulling with the remaining solution. Either way, you want to keep the oil in your mouth for a total of 15-20 minutes. Some people need to spit a portion of the oil out once, or even twice, before the end of the 20 minutes. That's okay.

Spit the oil into a trash receptacle or plastic bag. I do not recommend that you spit into the sink or the toilet, over time it could clog the drain. After spitting, rinse your mouth thoroughly with water to remove any residual oil. Your mouth and throat will probably feel very dry, so take a drink of water.

You can oil pull any time of the day. Ordinarily it is done at least once a day in the morning before eating breakfast. Oil pulling should be done on an empty stomach, especially if you are just beginning. Some people have a difficult time putting oil into their mouths because they are uncomfortable with the taste or the texture. As they pull, it may cause gagging, nausea, or possibly even vomiting, in which case you don't want a full stomach. After a few days of experience, you will get used to the oil and it will no longer bother you.

Most recommendations say to oil pull before eating or on an empty stomach (at least 3 to 4 hours after eating). This is important if you are just starting out. Once you have become familiar with oil pulling and feel comfortable with it, you can do it any time, even after a meal. The reason it is not recommended too soon after eating is that on a full stomach it is more likely to cause you to feel nauseated. Another reason is that the bacterial population in your mouth is at the highest level just before meals and at its lowest just after. When you eat, much of the bacteria are consumed and swallowed with your food. You remove more bacteria from your mouth if you pull before eating.

You may drink some water before oil pulling. This is actually recommended, especially if you have a dry mouth or feel dehydrated. Your body needs to be adequately hydrated in order to produce saliva, which is necessary for the oil pulling process. Saliva helps to remove and fight bacteria and balance pH.

In summary, the steps are as follows:

- Start on an empty stomach, a drink of water beforehand is okay and actually encouraged
- Take 2-3 teaspoons of liquid coconut oil into your mouth
- Suck, push, and pull the oil through the teeth and gums
- The solution will turn a milky white
- Swish the oil continually in the mouth for 15-20 minutes
- Discard the oil in the trash
- Rinse out the mouth and follow with a drink of water
- Follow this procedure at least once a day

Get into the habit of oil pulling at the same time every day, usually just after you get up in the morning and before eating breakfast. While you are oil pulling you can do other things to make effective use of your time. You can get dressed, take a shower, shave, put on make-up, make breakfast, read the paper, etc.

If you have an active infection in your mouth or another serious health problem, you can pull two, three, or more times a day to speed the healing process. Pulling just before meals is the best time because that way you won't forget.

If at first you have a hard time with the taste of the oil, you can add a few drops of cinnamon or peppermint oil to the coconut oil. This will also help freshen your breath. After you become comfortable with oil pulling, you can discontinue the flavored oils if you like.

At first it may seem difficult to work the oil for a full 20 minutes. When I first started oil pulling there were a few times I lost it. Mucous draining in the back of my throat, coughing, or sneezing, caused me to expel the contents of my mouth abruptly before finding a wastebasket. It can be messy. I learned to keep a cup or trashcan nearby just in case I needed to empty my mouth in a hurry. Now I've become more

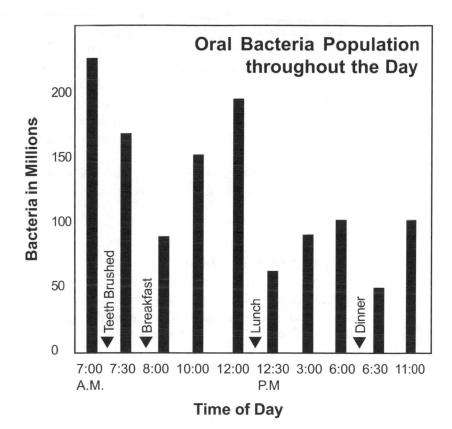

Oral Bacteria Population throughout the Day

Bacteria in Millions

200

150

100

50

0

Teeth Brushed

Breakfast

Lunch

Dinner

7:00 7:30 8:00 10:00 12:00 12:30 3:00 6:00 6:30 11:00
A.M.   P.M

Time of Day

This graph shows how the number of bacteria in the mouth changes throughout the day. In the process of eating, bacteria accumulate in the food and saliva and are eventually swallowed. Bacteria are greatest in number in the morning before breakfast. Brushing the teeth does not effectively remove bacteria. Teeth compose only 10 percent of the mouth, cleaning them thoroughly still leaves 90 percent of the mouth dirty. After brushing (7:30 a.m.), the number of bacteria remains high. After breakfast, bacteria increase in number almost to pre-breakfast levels (12:00 noon). Bacteria are at their lowest after eating dinner. As you sleep, bacteria have a chance to multiply without interruption. The lack of saliva secretion during sleep enhances bacteria growth. This is why it is important to oil pull first thing in the morning. Oil pulling before eating removes the greatest amount of bacteria and reduces the amount swallowed with food. (Source: L.W. Slanetz and E.A. Brown [2])

111

accustomed to having a mouthful of oil and I can clear my throat, cough, and sneeze without releasing any oil from my mouth.

Children as young as five years of age can do oil pulling. Depending on their age, give them 1-2 teaspoons, or whatever they feel comfortable using. Because a child's attention span is short, limit young children to 3-5 minutes. Flavored oil may make it easier for them. Make sure they spit the oil out and don't swallow it. The flavored oils can be tempting to swallow.

People report positive results from minor conditions in a matter of days. More serious problems may take several months or even a year or more.

WHAT OIL IS BEST FOR PULLING?

Dr. F. Karach mentions refined sunflower oil. Ayurvedic writings describing oil gargling, from which oil pulling was patterned, prescribe sesame oil. These oils are the most frequently mentioned in regard to oil pulling and were undoubtedly chosen because they are common household oils in India, where Ayurvedic medicine originated. Both oils work well, but *any* oil will work and just about any oil has been used.

Some people will claim, with no justification, that you must use either sunflower or sesame oil, or that the oils must be refined or organic and cold pressed, etc. The truth of the matter is that any oil will work and people have had good results using a variety of oils including olive oil, peanut oil, coconut oil, mustard oil, and even whole milk. Any of these will work, whether they are refined or unrefined, organic or not.

I personally prefer to use coconut oil, either virgin coconut oil or refined. The refined coconut oil is cheaper and, therefore, more economical. The reason for my choice is that I want to use a healthy oil, and coconut oil is by far healthier than sunflower, sesame oil, or any of these other vegetable oils. I also prefer an oil that has a mild taste, that is why Dr. Karach mentions *refined* sunflower oil. Many unrefined oils such as virgin olive oil and sesame oil have a strong flavor. Some brands of virgin coconut oil are strong too, but that is because of the processing. A good brand of virgin coconut oil has a mild, pleasant taste and the processed (also known as expeller pressed) coconut oil is essentially tasteless.

If you are not familiar with using coconut oil, you may be surprised to find that at room temperature it may be either liquid or solid. Coconut oil naturally has a high melting point. At 76 °F (24 °C) and above, it is a liquid, like most any other vegetable oil. Below this temperature it solidifies. All oils will do this at some temperature. Olive oil at room temperature is a liquid, but put it into the refrigerator and it will become solid.

I keep a jar of coconut oil on the countertop in my kitchen. During the summer it is often in a liquid state. During the winter it hardens. When I want to use it for oil pulling, I will put a spoonful into a small glass container and heat it on the stove for about a minute. It melts quickly.

WHAT TO EXPECT WHEN YOU BEGIN OIL PULLING
A Healing Crisis

Our mouths are the source of a large number of germs that eventually make their way into the rest of the body. The immune system can be overburdened fighting a continual battle against these invaders. When you begin oil pulling, you attack the source of these microscopic invaders and greatly reduce their numbers. This lifts a great deal of strain off the immune system and frees it up, so to speak, so that it can focus on cleaning house—detoxifying and healing the body. The immune system is now able to remove toxins and debris that may have been accumulating and affecting your health for years.

Oil pulling can have a powerful detoxing effect. Even with your first pull, you may experience heavy cleansing. Cleansing is generally most intense for the first few weeks. This makes sense, since at the beginning you have the greatest amount of accumulated microorganisms and toxins lodged in your mouth, throat, and sinuses. It may also make you feel queasy or nauseated. You may have to spit the oil out after just a few minutes because of mucous released in the throat that may initiate a gagging reaction. That's okay; clear your throat and take another spoonful of oil and keep at it for a total of 15-20 minutes.

After pulling, mucous may continue to drain from your throat and sinuses throughout the day. You may feel like you are coming down with a cold and may even have a "sore" throat. Don't worry. You are not getting sick; your body is just continuing the cleansing process initiated by the oil pulling.

As your body detoxifies, you may encounter any number of cleansing symptoms—sinus discharge, nausea, vomiting, diarrhea, skin outbreaks, aches and pains, headaches, fever, restlessness, fatigue, etc. Existing health problems such as joint pain, psoriasis, insomnia, and such may intensify for a time. Cleansing reactions normally only last a few days and at most a few weeks. Let the body complete the cleansing process without interruption. Continue oil pulling and avoid taking medication to treat the symptoms. Herbs and vitamins are generally okay because they don't interfere with the cleansing process. Drugs, for the most part, are chemicals foreign to the body and only burden the immune system with more debris to process and remove. They can slow down, and even stop, the healing process.

When cleansing reactions occur, this is called a *healing crisis*. It is referred to as a "crisis" because the symptoms can be discomforting. The healing crisis is beneficial. It is a sign that the body is healing itself. If you take drugs to stop the reaction, the healing process ends. For instance, if you are experiencing heavy mucous discharge, taking a decongestant will dry up the mucous. Toxins that were being expelled in the mucous now don't have a way to exit the body, so they remain entrenched inside your tissues.

The types of symptoms each person experiences from oil pulling will be different. One person may experience nasal congestion and headaches, another person may break out in a rash, and a third may have no noticeable symptoms at all, so you cannot predict what type of symptoms, if any, you may experience. We all have different genetic backgrounds, diets, lifestyles, and such, so our bodies will all react differently to any type of cleansing program.

Not everyone experiences unpleasant symptoms. Often the only noticeable reaction is a little excess mucous while oil pulling. Over time, as the body becomes cleaner and healthier, symptoms become less noticeable.

Sometimes when people experience a healing crisis they are confused. They mistakenly assume that oil pulling doesn't agree with them or it is making them sick. When they stop, the symptoms go away. They take this as proof that oil pulling is causing them harm.

They may claim that oil pulling didn't work for them or that it is even harmful. When you begin oil pulling you need to be aware that you may experience some unpleasant symptoms. Swishing vegetable oil in your mouth is *not* harmful in any way. It is the most benign, yet one of the most effective, natural methods of detoxification and cleansing.

For further understanding about the healing crisis, how to distinguish it from a disease crisis (illness), what to do and what not to do during a crisis, I highly recommend my book *The Healing Crisis* (see the bibliography at the end of this book).

Loose Fillings

Some people have reported that oil pulling loosened their dental fillings. The sucking and swishing action can dislodge loose fillings. Although this may sound bad, it is not a bad thing. If you lose a filling while oil pulling it means the filling was loose to begin with and, therefore, needed to come out. What made it loose? Either poor dentistry or continued tooth decay. In either case, it is best to have the filling replaced.

It is not just old fillings you need to worry about; even new fillings can come loose. If this happens, it means the dentist did a very poor job, as the fillings were not properly seated in the teeth. In time, bacteria would have seeped around and underneath the fillings and caused further decay, the eventual loss of the fillings, and possibly loss of the teeth.

If you have fillings that come out while oil pulling, this is really a blessing, especially if they are amalgams. This way you can replace them with safer composites. If the fillings are relatively new, don't go back to the same dentist for a replacement. If he or she couldn't put them in right the first time, it is not likely to be done correctly the next. Find a more competent dentist. Any filling that is loose enough to come out during oil pulling needs to come out before it causes serious problems.

HOW OIL PULLING WORKS

Oil pulling is one of the simplest, yet one of the most powerful, healing tools in natural medicine. To many people it is inconceivable that simply swishing oil in the mouth can have such a dramatic effect and can cure infections and debilitating degenerative disease. How does it work? How can oil placed in the mouth bring about such remarkable improvements in health?

The oil itself doesn't do the healing; it's the body that does that. All the oil does is provide a way for the body to heal itself. Our bodies are amazing organisms. We have, programmed within us, the ability to heal from just about any infectious or degenerative disease, if given the opportunity. By removing conditions that cause disease and providing your body with the things that it needs to rebuild and maintain good health, you can overcome just about any illness.

Oil pulling works by removing disease-causing microorganisms and toxins in the mouth that cause ill health. How does the oil work its magic? There is nothing magic about it; it is simple biology. Most of the microorganisms that inhabit the mouth consist of a single cell. These cells are covered with a lipid or fatty membrane, which is basically the cell's skin. Even the membranes surrounding our own cells are composed predominately of fat.

When you mix oil (fat) and water together, what happens? They separate. Oil and water do not mix. But when you add two oils together, what happens? They combine. They are attracted to each other. This is the secret to oil pulling. When you put oil into your mouth, the fatty membranes of the microorganisms are attracted to it. As you swish the oil around your teeth and gums, microbes are picked up as though they are being drawn to a powerful magnet. Bacteria hiding under crevices in the gums and in pores and tubules within the teeth are sucked out of their hiding places and held firmly in the solution. The longer you push and pull the oil though your mouth, the more microbes are pulled free. After 20 minutes the solution is filled with bacteria, viruses, and other organisms. This is why you want to spit it out rather than swallow it.

Food particles that get trapped between the teeth are also worked free. Much of it is also attracted to the oil, and if not, it is attracted to the saliva (water based) and still pulled out. So oil pulling literally "pulls" microbes and food particles (their food source) out of your mouth. The addition of saliva also helps to fight certain microbes and balances pH. Thus, you remove disease-causing substances and increase healing substances every time you pull. Without the burden of constantly fighting off oral infections and infiltrating bacteria and their toxins, the body is freed up to focus on self-healing. Inflammation is quieted, blood chemistry is normalized, damaged tissues are repaired, and healing occurs.

ORAL ECOLOGY

The types of microorganisms living in our mouths have a tremendous impact on our health. We all have basically the same types of organisms inhabiting our mouths. However, each person carries different proportions of these microbes. The inhabitants living in healthy mouths can be remarkably different from those living in diseased mouths. Certain bacteria increase in number, while others decrease. The higher the level of disease-causing bacteria, the more likely people are to have oral and systemic health problems. Reducing the number of troublesome microbes in the mouth reduces the risk of developing disease.

Bacteria and other microorganisms don't select our mouths, our mouths select them. The conditions in our mouths create an environment that favors certain types of organisms and allows them to grow and flourish. A healthy mouth (and healthy body) is filled with relatively benign bacteria for the most part. An unhealthy mouth attracts harmful bacteria. If you want to have a healthier mouth and body, you must change the environment in your mouth.

Researchers have tried various ways to alter the micro-populations in people's mouths. These populations can be altered *temporarily* by cleaning your teeth, using antiseptic mouthwashes, and even taking antibiotics. However, the ordinary inhabitants and their relative proportions to each other quickly reestablish themselves. Killing oral bacteria helps to reduce their numbers, but it does not change the types of organisms that thrive in the mouth.

So-called friendly organisms can inhibit or even kill the more troublesome ones. So increasing the number of good microbes would help lower the number of bad and keep them under control. This concept has proven useful for balancing the environment in the gut. Lactic acid bacteria in cultured foods like yogurt and sauerkraut, and probiotic dietary supplements help to build the populations of good bacteria and suppress the troublemakers, thus helping to relieve various digestive complaints.

117

This same concept has been tried with oral populations. Sigmund Socransky, an associate clinical professor of periodontology at Harvard, has been working with this concept. "We'd love to replace the bad guys with good guys," says Socransky. "That's being tried, but it turns out to be difficult." Socransky and colleagues put billions of beneficial bacteria in their own mouths and swished them around. But the good guys could not establish residence. So they packed the bacteria into a paste, which they rubbed on their teeth and gums. That didn't work either. Then Socransky saturated thick dental floss with bacteria, wrapped it around each tooth, and left it overnight. "Most of the bacteria we tried to introduce disappeared within four to five days," says Socransky.

Socransky's idea to increase good bacteria was correct, but his methods to accomplish it were all wrong. Like any ecological niche, it is the environment that determines what will and will not thrive there. For example, if you put a water-loving frog into a dry desert, the frog would soon wither up and die. The environment of the desert does not satisfy the frog's needs. No matter how may frogs you put into the desert, they are not going to survive.

Likewise, the ecology of the mouth isn't going to change simply because you introduce a certain type of organism. The environment in your mouth is established, for the most part, by your diet and lifestyle. In order to make permanent changes in the environment of your mouth, you need to make dietary and lifestyle changes.

Oil pulling works wonders for removing all types of germs and reducing the number of potentially harmful ones. But it is not a complete answer because it doesn't change the basic environment in the mouth which allows harmful bacteria to thrive. Oil pulling reduces the amount of total bacteria in our mouths, but it does not change the percentage of good to bad. This is why I developed my Oil Pulling Therapy program. It is designed to heal the mouth and the body by altering the oral ecology in a healthy, permanent way.

Chapter 7

Dr. Fife's
Oil Pulling Therapy

OIL PULLING THERAPY

I often hear people complain that they tried oil pulling, but it didn't do anything for them. Some people even claim that it made them worse! Why does it bring remarkable healing to some and yet for others appear to be worthless? Oil pulling is a useful technique, but it is not a cure-all. In fact, it's not a cure at all.

Oil pulling is a tool that is useful for removing harmful bacteria from the mouth. That is its purpose. If you have an active infection in the mouth, it can pull out the offending bacteria, giving the body the chance to heal itself. It is the body that brings about the cure, not the oil pulling. If the body does not heal, it is not because the oil pulling did not work, it is because your body was unable to do the healing.

Why wouldn't your body heal? There are many reasons. When you read the success stories of others, you can become overconfident and believe it will solve all your health problems overnight. This is unrealistic. If you have a health problem that may have taken 10 or 20 years to develop, you can't expect a cure overnight. Remember, oil pulling does not cure; it is the body that does the curing. It takes time for the body to heal itself. You would not expect a broken bone to heal itself in a few days or a week or two, so why would you expect something else to heal as quickly, especially a chronic degenerative condition that may have existed for many years? You have to be realistic.

Another reason why healing may not occur as quickly as expected is because you don't allow it to. If your body is sick due to poor dietary and lifestyle habits, you cannot expect to recover until you make changes. It is like hitting your thumb with a hammer. Putting a band-aid on it won't do any good if you keep on hitting it. Stop doing those things that cause damage to your health and allow the body to heal itself.

Oil pulling will do everything it is supposed to do, but if an illness is not related to oral health, it may not give you the results you expect. Not all health problems stem from oral infections. Illness can arise from an imbalance in the gut, an infected wound, sexual contact, genetic defect, or some other cause. Some of the same microorganisms that infect our mouths and wreak havoc in our bloodstream also live on the skin and in our environment and may enter the body in other ways. Even then, oil pulling can help by reducing stress on the immune system, so it can still be of great benefit.

My Oil Pulling Therapy program is more than just oil pulling. I transform oil pulling into a complete health-enhancing program that strengthens the immune system, fights off infection, enhances nutrient absorption, balances blood chemistry, and banishes health-destroying influences. The results are quicker, more complete, and more encompassing than what you get from oil pulling alone.

In the following sections each aspect of the program is discussed followed by a summary of the entire program at the end of the chapter.

HEALTHY DIET

Diet plays a central role in our health. The adage "you are what you eat" is very true. If you eat a diet loaded with junk foods, you will feel like garbage and your health will be in the dumps. Eating wholesome, nutrition-packed foods will provide you with the building blocks necessary to build and maintain a healthy body.

Most of us recognize the importance of eating healthfully; what most of us don't understand is what constitutes a healthy diet. Some people believe that if they eat a couple of servings of vegetables each day, they have a healthy diet. Others believe that if they cut out as much fat as possible, that is a healthy diet, regardless of what else they eat.

If you asked 10 people what they consider a healthy diet to be, you will get 10 different answers. Some will say a low-fat diet, others a low-carb diet, or Weight Watcher's, macrobiotics, or the Zone Diet, while others will say that vegetarianism is the way to go. Which of all these diets is the best? With new diets and new trends popping up all the time, people are confused. Many of these diets are designed specifically as a means for weight loss. A weight-loss diet is not necessarily the healthiest, nor may it be one you would want to live on for the rest of your life. The same thing applies to detox diets. They are designed to quickly cleanse the body but are not suitable for long term use. Who would want to remain on a vegetable juice diet all their life? These diets can serve useful purposes, but in the long run you need a diet that is packed with nutrition, shy on calories, and yet tasteful and satisfying.

There are many conflicting opinions about which foods and diets are good and which are bad. You can't trust the so-called experts because they can't agree themselves. Some say saturated fat, cholesterol, and red meat are bad, while other say they are good, it's the sugar and processed grains that are bad, and so forth. What are you to believe? There is an answer.

You can study nutritional science and theorize about diets all you want, but the real test is to see which ones work in the real world. Theories are fine, but if they don't work, they're no good. A healthy diet is one that strengthens the body, making it capable of fighting off disease and maintaining good health throughout life and into old age. Our current, so-called Western diet is sadly lacking. Despite reducing cholesterol, cutting down on saturated fat, and other measures, degenerative diseases are rising to all time highs, and new diseases are constantly appearing. Diseases that at one time were considered afflictions of old age, such as adult-onset diabetes (type 2) and arthritis, are occurring at younger and younger ages. Current dietary guidelines are a disaster. So what's the answer?

The key to finding the ideal diet is to look at populations that have a low incidence of degenerative disease, including tooth decay and gum disease. A population cannot be healthy on a poor diet. Therefore, healthy populations have healthy diets. Today it is hard to find such populations. With international trade, modern Western foods are available worldwide. Consequently, heart disease, cancer, diabetes, and other degenerative diseases now plague the entire world.

At the beginning of the twentieth century, however, there were many populations around the world who had not yet been exposed to modern foods and were unaffected by the so-called diseases of modern civilization. Thanks to the pioneering work of Dr. Weston A. Price, we have records of healthy societies and the foods they ate. It was Dr. Price who compiled the most extensive research on focal infections in the 1920s. In the years that followed, he also discovered the link between degenerative disease and diet.

During Dr. Price's long career as a practicing dentist, he observed the growing number of people who were developing degenerative diseases and dental problems. He was seeing an increasing number of dental conditions late in his career that were rare in his earlier years. During the early part of the twentieth century food production and processing was revolutionized in order to meet demands for a rapidly growing population.

The invention of the hydraulic press and the hydrogenation of vegetable oils changed the types of oils and fats in the diet. Before the 1920s animal fats and tropical oils were the predominate sources of fat in the diet. Vegetable seed oils were not used much because of the difficulty and expense of extracting the oil from seeds. The hydraulic press simplified the process making vegetable oils less expensive than animal fats. Hydrogenation transformed cheap vegetable oils into hard fats that could replace the more expensive animal fats. Lard and butter gave way to vegetable shortening and margarine.

Sugar and flour production became more automated. From 1900 to 1930 sugar consumption increased 10-fold. White bread became the mainstay in the diet. Bread became lighter, softer, and with the aid of preservatives would last longer without spoiling. Jellies, jams, canned goods, and sweets of all types started filling grocery store shelves. Preservatives, flavor enhances, artificial dyes, and other chemicals were added to processed foods. Raw milk, the standard throughout all of history, was now pasteurized and homogenized. The era of modern food production had begun. The American diet and, in fact, the diet of the entire Western world, began to make a dramatic change.

As food processing evolved and the diet changed, an interesting phenomenon also began to occur. It was so subtle that few took notice, but otherwise rare or unheard of diseases began to increase in number. Coronary heart disease, which was almost unheard of before the 1920s, exploded on the scene and by the 1950s became the nation's number one cause of death. It is interesting that today animal fats and cholesterol are often blamed for causing heart disease, yet at the turn of the twentieth century when animal fats were the primary source of fat in the diet and saturated fat and cholesterol consumption were much higher than they are now, heart disease was rare.

Dr. Price was a witness to the dramatic shift in diet and the rise of dental and degenerative diseases. He wondered if the changes in the diet were related to the decline in health. He set out to find the answer. The way he planned to do this was to compare the health of people who ate traditional diets with those who ate modern processed foods. To avoid other influences that may affect health, the people studied would be of the same genetic background and live in the same geographic area. The only difference would be the diet.

Today it is nearly impossible to find a population that relies solely on traditional foods. Modern foods are found virtually everywhere throughout the world. But in the 1930s there were still many populations that subsisted primarily on their ancestral foods without modern influences.

Dr. Price spent nearly a decade traveling around the world locating and studying these populations. He traveled to isolated valleys in the Swiss Alps, the Outer and Inner Hebrides off the coast of Scotland, visited Eskimo villages in Alaska, American Indians in Central and Northern Canada and in Florida, the Melanesians and Polynesians on numerous islands in the South Pacific, tribes in eastern and central Africa, The Aborigines of Australia, Malay tribes on islands north of Australia, the Maori of New Zealand, and South American Indians in Peru and the Amazon Basin.

When Dr. Price visited an area, he would examine the people's health, particularly their teeth, and made careful note of the foods they ate, meticulously analyzing the nutritional content of the diet. Samples of the foods were sent to his laboratory where detailed analyses were made. It didn't take long for him to notice the contrast in health between those who lived entirely on indigenous foods and those who had incorporated Western foods into their diets.

Wherever he found people living on traditional foods, he noted that both their dental and physical health were in excellent condition, but when the people began eating modern foods, their health declined. In the absence of modern medical care, physical degeneration was pronounced. Dental diseases, as well as infectious and degenerative diseases such as arthritis and tuberculosis, were common among those eating Western foods. For instance, the differences between Pacific islanders who lived inland and those who lived near the ports, where modern foods were available, were readily apparent (see photos on page 125). Speaking of the inland inhabitants Dr. Price noted, "The physical development of the primitive people, including their teeth and dental arches is of very high order. A comparison of the individuals living near the ports with those living in the isolated inland locations shows marked increase in the incidence of dental caries. For those living almost exclusively on the native foods the incidence of dental caries was only 0.14 tenths of a percent, while for those using trade foods the incidence of dental caries was 26 percent." He went on to observe that there was also a "progressive development of degenerative diseases around the port."[1]

It didn't take a dramatic change in the diet for degenerative disease to begin to creep in. Simply adding a few commercial products, which displaced more nutritious foods, was all that was needed. The most common imported foods were white flour, polished rice, sugar, vegetable oils, and canned goods.

Of the groups Dr. Price studied, the average number of teeth affected by cavities among those who ate traditional foods was only 0.79 percent (less than 8 out of every 1,000 teeth examined) while the number of cavities in those who ate Western foods was over 33 percent (333 out of 1,000 teeth). Among those eating modern foods, 90-100 percent of them suffered from dental cavities. Those who ate traditional diets had much better dental health despite the fact that they did not brush their teeth, floss, use whiteners or disinfectant mouthwashes, or get any professional dental care. Their good dental health was a direct

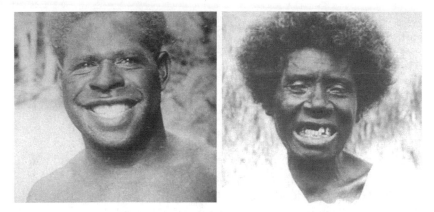

South Pacific Islanders. Left: Shows a young man of one of the Malay tribes who splendidly illustrates magnificent facial and dental arch development. Right: In contrast, we see a Melanesian woman who lives at a port where modern foods are received and used liberally. Her beauty is lost through tooth decay. Photos taken by Dr. Weston A. Price. Copyright Price-Pottenger Nutrition Foundation, www.ppnf.org.

result of eating healthy foods. Dental health clearly mirrored their physical health.

Dr. Price's findings were published in 1939 in a book titled *Nutrition and Physical Degeneration*. This book, which is still in print and currently in its eighth edition, is considered a classic in nutritional science.

One of the interesting things that came from Dr. Price's work was that all of the traditional diets that he studied were effective in protecting the people from dental decay and providing them with good health. It was only after they began to abandon their traditional diets for modern foods that dental and physical health declined. This is interesting because these traditional diets were very different from one another. Some were very high in saturated fat, meat, or milk, while others were low in these foods but high in fruits, vegetables, or grains. Some ate fish; some ate no fish. Some had a high vegetable diet while others ate no vegetables or fruits whatsoever, relying totally on meat and milk. The types of vegetables, fruits, and grains all differed, but

125

they were all *whole* foods, not processed. Sugar and refined carbohydrate consumption was nonexistent. Processed vegetable oil consumption was nonexistent; they ate coconut oil, butter, and animal fat, and in many cases, lots of it. They consumed no packaged, commercially processed, or convenience foods. Everything was homemade.

From Dr. Price's research we learn that it is not the type of food that is important, but rather what we do to the food that makes the difference. In other words, the best diet consists entirely of whole organic foods. Nothing commercially processed or prepared. When you go shopping for food, focus on buying whole foods that are fresh, dried, frozen, or fermented. Most of your diet should consist of fresh fruits and vegetables, whole grains (make you own bread), fresh organic meats, fats, and raw and fermented dairy. As a basic rule of thumb, if a food is sold in a can, package, or box, then it is best not to eat it.

I am aware that not everyone is willing to prepare everything they eat from scratch. Avoiding all commercially prepared foods is difficult, especially if you have a social life and have little control over which foods you are offered. You have to decide how strict you want to be.

There are some food products that are definitely more troublesome than others. If you do eat some processed foods, the ones you need to avoid the most are sugary foods and drinks, refined grains, and processed vegetable oils. While it won't kill you to eat these products once in awhile, keep in mind that the more of them you eat, the closer you will come to experiencing tooth decay, gum disease, and physical degeneration.

THE SUGAR CURSE

I like cake, ice cream, and candy—who doesn't? There have been times I would eat a cookie or some other treat and immediately want another, and another, until I'd consumed far too much. It's like an addiction. You can't eat just one. Sugar stimulates pleasure centers in the brain, much like cocaine, and can be just about as addictive. In fact, studies show that when lab animals are given the choice between sugar and cocaine, they prefer the sugar!

Tooth Decay Through History

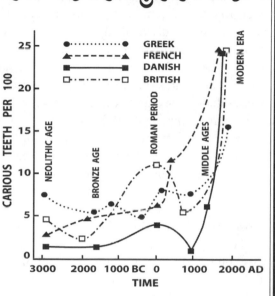

Cavities and gum disease were rare among prehistoric humans. In the most ancient hominids, the incidence of cavities is less than 1 percent. Dr. Weston A. Price found that modern societies that lived solely on traditional foods had about the same cavity rate. Among those eating modern foods, the rate was typically 20-40 percent and as high as 70 percent.

The incidence of cavities in Europe was relatively low throughout most of history and began to increase dramatically during the Middle Ages when sugarcane became accessible to the Western world.

Source: University of Illinois at Chicago

Refined sugar is perhaps the most detrimental food in our diet. Refined carbohydrates, such as white flour and polished white rice, are not much better because they are quickly converted into sugar in our digestive tracts and have much of the same adverse effects.

Sugar in itself is not bad, in fact, our cells use sugar as a source of energy. It is the excess consumption of sugar and refined carbohydrates that causes the problem. Much of our diet consists of both simple and

127

complex carbohydrates. Sugar is a carbohydrate—a simple carbohydrate. It is the basic building block for all carbohydrates. Complex carbohydrates are nothing more than long chains of sugar molecules linked together. During the process of digestion, enzymes break the links, releasing individual sugar molecules, which are then absorbed into the bloodstream to be used as food for our cells. Fiber is also a complex carbohydrate, but it is structured in such a way that the body cannot break the links between the sugar molecules, so it is not absorbed. It passes though the digestive tract mostly intact. Complex carbohydrates are the main components of fruits, vegetables, grains, nuts, and seeds.

When you eat foods containing complex carbohydrates, sugars are released slowly and enter the bloodstream at a relatively constant rate. This allows time for the pancreas to produce insulin, which pulls the sugar from the bloodstream and shuttles it into the cells where it is utilized to produce energy. However, when you eat pure sugar, it goes almost immediately into the bloodstream.

The average sized adult has about 1.5 gallons (5.6 liters) of blood in his or her body. In that gallon and a half of blood, a healthy individual will have the equivalent of about 1-3 teaspoons of sugar. When you eat a 2.2-ounce Snickers candy bar, which contains the equivalent of 9 teaspoons of sugar, or a cup of vanilla ice cream with 8 teaspoons of sugar, or a slice of apple pie with 10 teaspoons, you are pumping a large amount of sugar all at once into your bloodstream. Blood sugar levels rise dramatically. If your blood sugar rises too high or remains elevated for too long, you will go into a hyperglycemic coma and die. Excess blood sugar is toxic to your body. The higher the sugar content the greater the harm. Your body works frantically to prevent damage by producing insulin to keep blood sugar at appropriate levels. This reaction keeps you from dying when you eat sugar, but high levels of insulin are also toxic. The more often you consume excessive amounts of sugar the greater your risk of developing health problems such as high blood pressure (which promotes heart disease), diabetes, and obesity.

One of the major consequences of eating sugar is a reduction in your ability to fight off infection. Sugar depresses immune function, allowing microbes to multiply and spread through the body. I work with a person who is always coming into the office with nasal congestion, sniffles, and coughing. It seems like he is sick more often than not. He is always eating candy and I think that is his problem. He doesn't like to eat vegetables but loves sweets and eats them every day. His wife and family have taken on his eating habits and they too are just as sick as he is. Every time I see his family, one of them is always sick. After speaking with a doctor, he decided to cut back on his candy intake. The result was dramatic. He was able to function for several weeks straight without constantly sniffing and choking on mucous.

Another problem with sugar is that it provides no nutritional benefit other than calories. Sugar is a source of empty calories. Most of us can do with fewer calories in our diet. Sugar supplies no useful nutrients, however, vitamins and minerals are consumed when sugar is processed in the body, thus decreasing nutrient reserves. Not only does it deplete nutrients, but when you eat foods loaded with sugar, you displace other more nutritious foods from your diet. Excess sugar consumption, therefore, promotes malnutrition, which in turn, also lowers immune function.

The reason dentists don't like sugar is because it rots the teeth. As mentioned earlier, sugar feeds acid-producing bacteria which cause tooth decay. Every time you eat sugary foods, or refined carbohydrates, you are feeding the bacteria that rot your teeth and pave the way for oral and systemic infection. The more often you eat sugary foods, the more often you feed teeth-killing bacteria.

Sodas, candy, and desserts are the worst things you can consume. The sugar content is so high that it is like putting fertilizer on the bacteria in your mouth. The sugar reaches every crack and cranny in your mouth, igniting a feeding frenzy and a surge of bacteria growth and acid production.

If you are going to eat sweets, it is better to eat them all at one time and with meals than it is to spread them out over the day. That way the sugar is only in the mouth for a limited amount of time. If you need to snack on something between meals, it is best not to eat sweets. Eat real food instead, like vegetables, meat, cheese, or anything without sugar or refined carbohydrates. Crackers, bread, chips, and such that are made with white flour aren't much better than sugar. White flour is easily broken down into sugar by salivary enzymes.

Our teeth are porous, especially the dentin with its numerous tubules. Nutrient-rich fluids flow from the roots of the teeth outward through the tubules. The normal flow of this fluid is from the inside of the tooth to the outside. When we eat sugar, however, the flow of this fluid reverses, going inwards toward the root. This poses a big problem. When fluid flow goes into the tooth, it carries with it sugar and bacteria. This allows bacteria to infiltrate inside the teeth where they can establish colonies. Every time you eat sugar, you bring in food for these acid-producing bacteria to live on. In time, they will rot out the center of the teeth. A tooth can look normal on the outside, but inside can be hollowed out by decay.

In many ways, the chemistry of your saliva reflects the chemistry of your blood. Every time you eat sugar, your blood sugar level rises. Likewise, the sugar level in your saliva also rises. Sugar in your saliva feeds bacteria. So after eating sugar, even if you carefully rinse your mouth and brush your teeth, it won't make much difference because the sugar will come right back through your saliva.

If you are pre-diabetic or diabetic, this is of particular concern. In diabetes blood sugar levels rise higher and remain elevated longer than normal. For this reason, diabetics are particularly vulnerable to tooth decay. Tooth decay and gum disease cause infections that can seep into the bloodstream, which can cause systemic inflammation, leading to a rise in blood sugar. As blood sugar increases, so do salivary sugars, feeding the bacteria that promote gum disease. Thus you have a vicious circle. Gum disease promotes diabetes and diabetes promotes gum disease. The solution is simple: avoid eating sugar and refined carbohydrates.

DIETARY OILS

Of all the foods we eat, none have been as misrepresented and misunderstood as the dietary oils. Saturated fats have been demonized and polyunsaturated fats have been given sainthood, based primarily on the fact that the latter reduces blood cholesterol in comparison to the former. This concept has been promoted and kept alive by promoters of the cholesterol theory of heart disease, in other words, the pharmaceutical industry and their friends. In truth, saturated fats are the good guys and polyunsaturated fats the fiends.

The dominant fat in the diets of *all* the healthy people Dr. Weston A. Price studied was saturated, yet heart disease was absent among them. Disease attacked those who had abandoned their traditional diets, exchanging saturated fat for processed vegetable oils and other modern foods. This was seen in every population he studied throughout his travels around the world. The African Masai, Canadian Indians, and Alaskan Eskimos, whose diets consisted almost entirely of saturated fat and meat, were free from heart disease, yet once they began to eat processed oils and other modern foods, their health rapidly declined.

Many of Melanesians and Polynesians in the South Pacific Islands ate a diet high in saturated fat from coconuts. Some populations consumed up to 50 percent of their daily calories as saturated fat. Again, they were healthy and free from heart and other degenerative diseases. These diseases crept in after modern foods were introduced.

Although processed vegetable oils (safflower, corn, soybean, sunflower, cottonseed, etc.) have been promoted as being healthy, they are far from it. Compared to saturated fats, they are very unstable and go rancid quickly. This is why they are not commonly used in baked goods and other prepared foods. When heated, as in cooking foods, polyunsaturated oils degrade rapidly, generating harmful free radicals. Saturated fats are much more stable and are healthier to use for cooking.

All processed polyunsaturated oils have undergone some degree of oxidation by the time you buy them in the store. As soon as seeds are crushed and the oil is exposed to oxygen, heat, or light, oxidization begins. When oxidation occurs, free radicals are formed and the oil starts to go rancid. Oxidation continues as the oil is refined, bottled, transported, and stored on the store shelf and in your own kitchen. If you use the oil in cooking, oxidization is greatly accelerated, making it even more rancid and unhealthy.

Free radicals cause systemic inflammation and tissue degradation. Free radicals destroy cell walls and even DNA, leading to cellular death and cancer. In fact, polyunsaturated vegetables oils are well known for their cancer-causing effects.[2] Studies show that when cancer is chemically induced in animals, the type of fat in their diet determines

131

the number and size of the resulting tumors. Polyunsaturated fats produce the greatest number and the largest tumors. Monounsaturated fats, like olive oil, produce fewer, and saturated fats the least. Of the saturated fats, coconut oil has shown to produce the least number of tumors; in fact, coconut oil can completely prevent tumor development, even when the animals are given very potent cancer-causing chemicals.[3-5] Coconut oil is a powerful anti-cancer food.

Processed vegetable oils also depress the immune system. This fact is so well known that vegetable oil emulsions with water are given as intravenous injections for the purpose of suppressing immunity in patients who have had organ transplants.[6] One of the ways unsaturated fats hinder the immune system is by killing white blood cells. White blood cells, which defend us against harmful microorganisms, are the primary component of our immune system. If you are trying to rid yourself of systemic and oral infections, you certainly don't want to use something that lowers the efficiency of your immune system, or, for that matter, promotes inflammation and cancer.

Coconut oil would be a far better choice. It has anti-inflammatory and immune-enhancing properties as well as being anti-cancerous. Coconut oil has many other benefits; it protects against heart disease, liver disease, kidney disease, IBS, diabetes, and helps balance hormone levels.[7] Perhaps its most remarkable characteristic is its ability to kill disease-causing bacteria, viruses, fungi, and protozoa.

Among the dietary fats, coconut oil is unique because it is composed of a special group of fat molecules known as medium chain fatty acids (MCFAs). The only other food in the human diet that has any appreciable amount of MCFAs is breast milk. These special fats are essential for the health of newborn infants and are added to scientifically designed infant formulas. These unique fatty acids have many important uses. They are very easy to digest, providing a quick and easy source of nutrition, which is important to infants. They also possess powerful antimicrobial properties, so are capable of killing disease-causing microbes, which is essential for infants. In fact, it is primarily the presence of MCFAs in human breast milk that protects newborn babies from infections for the first few months of life while their immune systems are still developing. The fatty acids that protected us as infants also protect us as adults when we eat coconut oil.

Coconut oil's fatty acids kill many of the same types of bacteria and viruses that inhabit the mouth and cause infections elsewhere in the body. Antibiotics can kill bacteria, but they are useless against viruses. There are no drugs that can effectively kill viruses, but MCFAs can. They also kill yeasts and fungi, including candida. MCFAs aren't a universal remedy for all infections, however. They don't kill all bacteria, which is actually a good thing. They don't harm the friendly bacteria in our gut, so they don't cause digestive disturbances. Coconut oil can help clear the gut of harmful organisms, while leaving the harmless or beneficial ones alone.

Coconut helps keep teeth healthy. Even eating coconut meat, which contains the oil, can help to promote good dental health. In the coastal areas of northern Brazil, where coconuts are commonly consumed, the incidence of tooth decay and gum disease are reportedly lower than in other parts of the country. Even the poor, who don't have access to the best dental or health care, have healthier mouths than the more affluent non-coconut eaters.

This same observation was made by Dr. Weston A. Price when he studied the peoples in the South Pacific islands. Those people who maintained their traditional coconut-based diet had extraordinarily good dental health. He reported that they had a cavity rate of only 0.34 percent. That means out of every 1,000 teeth examined, he found only 3.4 teeth with cavities. Gum disease was essentially absent. In comparison, we have at least 10 times this many cavities and most of us have some level of gum disease.

For optimal health benefit, I recommend that you consume between 1-3 tablespoons of coconut daily as a part of your normal diet. Use coconut oil in place of other oils, especially processed vegetable oils, in food preparation. In recipes that call for vegetable oil, margarine, or shortening, use coconut oil instead. Coconut oil is very heat-stable and does not form free radicals like other vegetable oils do, so it makes an excellent cooking oil. You can also take the oil by the spoonful like a dietary supplement, as many people do. A good quality virgin coconut oil has a pleasant taste, and processed coconut oils have essentially no taste, so taking them by the spoonful isn't really difficult.

Because of coconut oil's antimicrobial effects, its ability to enhance the healing of injuries, and its many other health-promoting properties,

I recommend coconut oil for oil pulling. Why use any other inferior oil, when you can use coconut oil?

FLUID CONSUMPTION

One important aspect of good dental health is proper hydration—consuming adequate amounts of water. Dehydration results when the body loses excess body fluids. Dehydration may not seem like much of a problem, but it is far more serious and widespread than you might think. Water is essential for all chemical reactions in the body and a deficiency can seriously affect body function. A loss of just 1 percent of the body's fluids interferes with heat regulation and impairs mental and physical performance. A loss of as little as 8-10 percent can lead to a coma and death. By the time you "feel" thirsty you are already substantially dehydrated. Most of us do not drink enough water and walk around every day in a state of chronic subclinical dehydration—underhydration without obvious symptoms.

The general recommendation to maintain proper hydration is to drink six to eight glasses of water a day. A study by the National Research Council revealed that on average, women (ages 15-49) drink a mere 2.6 cups of water a day.[8] This finding suggests that a large portion of women may be chronically dehydrated. Another study carried out at Johns Hopkins Hospital in Baltimore discovered that 32-41 percent of the subjects they tested (both men and women ages 23-44) were chronically dehydrated.[9] Food consumption surveys indicate that as much as 75 percent of the population (all ages) may be chronically mildly dehydrated.

How does dehydration affect oral health? One of the most prominent symptoms of dehydration is dry mouth. As the body becomes dehydrated, saliva secretion decreases. Adequate saliva production is

---

"In the absence of salivation, the oral tissues become ulcerated and otherwise infected, and caries of the teeth become rampant."
Arthur C. Guyton, M.D., *Textbook of Medical Physiology*

---

essential for maintaining pH, fighting off certain harmful microorganisms, and maintaining a healthy oral environment. When you become dehydrated, your mouth is one of the first things to suffer. Chronic subclinical dehydration can significantly affect the environment in your mouth, altering microbial populations in an unhealthy way.

Many of us don't drink the recommended six to eight glasses of water during the day. Often people rely on coffee or soda for their daily fluid allowance. These types of beverages are no substitute for water. They can actually have a dehydrating effect, so your need for water increases. As a general rule of thumb, for every cup of coffee, tea, or soda you drink, you need to drink at least half that much again in water. So if you drink four cups of coffee per day, you need to drink an additional two cups of plain water to equal the fluid intake you would get from just four cups of water. Alcohol dries up the body big time. For every ounce of alcohol you consume, you need to drink an additional 5.5 ounces of water.

How much water do you need? We often hear the recommendation of six to eight glasses a day. One glass holds 12 ounces of water. The amount of water you need depends on your size. A large person needs more water than a smaller person. A general rule of thumb is to drink one glass (12 ounces) of water for every 25 pounds (12 kg) of bodyweight. A 100-pound person, therefore, needs to drink at least four glasses (48 ounces) of water a day. A 200-pound person needs eight glasses (96 ounces).

The healthiest fluid to consume is pure, clean water without flavorings, additives, chlorine, or fluoride. To avoid chlorine and fluoride you need to use some type of water filter or purifier that can remove these chemicals. If you want flavored water, add a squeeze of lemon or lime juice.

Coconut water is another good, natural source of fluids. Coconut water is the fluid from inside coconuts. It is rich in potassium and other minerals and contains only about a fifth as much sugar as most fruit juices and soft drinks. Coconut water is an excellent beverage for keeping hydrated because it contains essential electrolytes (ionic minerals) that are lost as we become dehydrated. Coconut water has gained popularity as a "natural" sports rehydration beverage and actually rehydrates the body better than plain water or commercial sports drinks.[10]

VITAMINS AND MINERALS

A good diet will supply most of the vitamins and minerals you need to be healthy. However, there are some important nutrients that are not normally consumed in optimal quantities. Taking vitamin and mineral dietary supplements can help boost your immune system, strengthen bones and teeth, improve oral health, alkalize your body (and saliva), and aid in your quest for better overall health.

One of the most important nutrients for good oral health is vitamin C. Unlike most animals, the humans cannot make their own vitamin C. We get vitamin C from eating fruits and vegetables. Vitamin C is a water-soluble vitamin and, as such, is not stored to any appreciable amount in the body. Therefore, we need to consume the vitamin every day. This means eating *fresh* fruits and vegetables daily. Cooking destroys vitamin C so packaged foods are usually deficient in this important nutrient.

Vitamin C performs many essential functions in the body. It is necessary for the production of collagen. Collagen is a connective tissue that holds our bodies together, including the connective tissues around the teeth, and provides the underlying framework on which bone and teeth are formed. Symptoms of vitamin C deficiency include bleeding gums, loosened teeth, bone fragility, spontaneous bruising, failure of wounds to heal, anemia, and muscle degeneration. Notice how many of these symptoms affect oral health? A deficiency in vitamin C can set the stage for serious dental problems.

Severe vitamin C deficiency manifests itself as scurvy, a potentially lethal disease. Many people do not eat adequate amounts of fresh produce and although they may not develop full-blown scurvy, they can have a mild or subclinical vitamin C deficiency. A mild deficiency is still a serious problem and can adversely affect gum health. Studies show that bleeding and inflammation varies directly with changes in vitamin C intake.[11]

The recommended dietary allowance (RDA) for vitamin C in the US and Canada is set at 60 mg per day. This is enough to prevent a

136

full-blown case of scurvy, but not necessarily enough to prevent a subclinical deficiency. Vitamin C is involved in the process of internal detoxification and in immune system function. In times of sickness, stress, or when exposed to smog or other toxins, our need for vitamin C greatly increases. In our daily lives we are constantly coming into contact with potentially harmful germs, experience loads of stress, and are exposed to all types of environmental toxins and pollutants, so our real need for vitamin C is much greater than the established RDA. Long-time vitamin C advocate and two-time Nobel Prize recipient Dr. Linus Pauling advocated taking much larger quantities, up to 4,000 mg a day. This recommendation was not simply to prevent deficiency, but to take advantage of the multitude of health benefits afforded by vitamin C. For similar reasons, and for the fact that vitamin C is so essential to the health of the teeth and gums, I recommend taking at least 500-1000 mg daily.

Vitamins A and D are necessary in the modeling and mineralizing of the bones. A deficiency in either can cause bones and teeth to become soft. Vitamin D deficiency, for example, leads to rickets in children and osteomalacia in adults. Vitamin D is known as the sunshine vitamin because it can be manufactured in our skin upon activation from direct sunlight. Getting adequate sunlight every day is the best source of vitamin D. Most of us, however, don't get enough sun exposure. In the winter, when the sun's rays are less intense, it can be near impossible to get enough sun to produce the needed vitamin D. Studies show that most people who live and work indoors are vitamin D deficient. This is, without a doubt, one of the reasons why many people in Western countries, regardless of calcium intake, experience a great deal of bone loss as they age. In fact, people in Third World countries who eat far less calcium, but get much more sun exposure, have much stronger bones. The RDA for vitamin D is 400 IU. Your body can make this amount with about 30 minutes of bright sun exposure. In the winter the time needed may be significantly greater.

The teeth are a part of our skeletal system and soft bones means soft teeth. In order to have strong, dense, healthy teeth, you need to have strong, dense, healthy bones. The same materials that build bone also build teeth. When we think of bone, we automatically think of calcium. Calcium is the primary mineral in our bones and we need adequate amounts of this mineral in order to have strong bones and teeth. Calcium, however, isn't the only mineral in bone. You can eat two, three, or four times the RDA of calcium but it won't do you any good if you don't have the other vitamins and minerals necessary for bone formation. Without adequate vitamin D, for instance, your bones become soft and weak, and taking calcium supplements won't do you any good. Other minerals needed for healthy bone formation include phosphorous, magnesium, boron, sulfur, zinc, manganese, and silica.

Unfortunately there has been too much emphasis on calcium and not enough on the other nutrients, which are just as important. The RDA of calcium in the US is set at 1,200 mg per day. This is more than adequate; in fact, it is probably too much. Many people get far less calcium than this yet have strong bones into old age. The World Health Organization (WHO) recommends only 400-500 mg daily. This is a more reasonable amount. Western diets have ample sources of calcium from milk, cheese, yogurt, seafood, green vegetables, legumes, supplements, and a wide variety of foods fortified with extra calcium.

Getting enough calcium isn't a problem. A bigger problem is getting adequate amounts of magnesium. The dietary intake of magnesium in North America and Europe is in general about half the recommended 420 mg for men and 320 mg for women. The best dietary sources are leafy greens, legumes, nuts, and seeds—foods of which we generally don't eat enough.

Calcium and magnesium act as antagonists, consequently, too much of one can cause a deficiency in the other, or too little of one can cause an excess in the other. They need to be in balance. At current recommendations the ratio of calcium to magnesium is about three-to-one. However, research by Guy Abraham, M.D. and Harinder Grewal, M.D. has demonstrated that the ideal ratio of calcium to magnesium is closer to one-to-one.[12]

They recorded significant increases (11 percent) in bone density in postmenopausal subjects when they were given only 500 mg of calcium and increased magnesium to 600 mg. In comparison, taking the RDA levels of calcium and magnesium after menopause does not improve bone density.

Excess calcium can cause high blood calcium levels, which can lead to calcium being deposited in parts of the body where it doesn't

Important Nutrients for Oral Health

Vitamin/Mineral	US RDA	Recommended
Vitamin A	1,000 RE	
Vitamin B1 (Thiamin)	1.5 mg	
Vitamin B2 (Riboflavin)	1.7 mg	
Vitamin B3 (Niacin)	20 mg	
Vitamin B6	2.0 mg	
Vitamin B12	6 mcg	
Vitamin C	60 mg	500-1000 mg
Vitamin D	400 IU	
Vitamin E	30 IU	200-400 IU
Folate	0.4 mg	
Calcium	1,200 mg	400-600 mg
Magnesium	400 mg	400-600 mg
Selenium	70 mcg	
Pantothenic acid	10 mg*	
Biotin	30 mcg*	
Chromium	50-200 mcg*	
Copper	2.0 mg*	
Manganese	5.0 mg*	
Molybdenum	250 mcg*	
Zinc	15 mg	
Iodine	150 mcg	
Lipoic acid	50-100 mg*	
CoQ10	10-30 mg*	
Boron	3-5 mg*	

*No RDA established. Values listed are estimated safe and adequate maintenance doses.

Take at least the Recommended Dietary Allowance (RDA) each day, except as noted under the "Recommended" column. You can benefit from a supplement that contains other nutrients that are not listed here. Use a supplement or combination of supplements that supply as many nutrients on this list as possible.

belong, such as the kidneys (stones), surface of the bone (bone spurs), arteries (atherosclerosis), and perhaps even teeth (tarter). Limiting calcium supplementation and increasing magnesium consumption can put calcium where it belongs.

Since calcium consumption is typically too high and magnesium consumption too low, many people have a calcium/magnesium imbalance. Multiple vitamin and mineral supplements are often not helpful because they provide too much calcium and not enough magnesium. It is recommended that you add about 200-400 mg of magnesium *without* added calcium. If you take a calcium supplement, limit it to no more than about 400-600 mg and increase total magnesium intake to 400-600 mg so that your ratio is one-to-one. Abraham and Grewal used a calcium-to-magnesium ratio of five-to-six, and suggest a ratio of one-to-two might even be better. A little more magnesium may be best to offset the higher calcium content normally found in the diet.

Adding magnesium to the diet can cause loose stools. If this happens, cut back on the dose. Over time as your body adjusts to the added magnesium, you can try increasing the amount you take. Better yet, add more magnesium-rich foods to your diet.

Next to calcium, phosphorus is the most abundant mineral in the human body. About 85 percent of the phosphorus is located in our bones and teeth. Our dietary requirement for phosphorus is about the same as that for calcium. Ideally, we should have a one-to-one ratio of calcium to phosphorus. Phosphorus is normally abundant in the diet. Meat, dairy, and eggs are rich sources. Several trace elements are also important in maintaining bone health. Boron, sulfur, zinc, manganese, and silica are only minor structural components of teeth and bone, but they play important functional roles in bone metabolism and bone turnover.

If you suffer from chronic illness, your immune system is probably overworked and the likelihood of a vitamin or mineral deficiency is high. Taking nutritional supplements could be of great help in your search for better health. Page 137 lists some of the major nutrients necessary for good health. You should get at least the RDA amounts of most of these; the exception is calcium, where a lower value is recommended. In some cases the RDA is inadequate, so a higher value is recommended. Your health care provider may also recommend higher amounts of certain nutrients for specific health conditions.

DENTAL CARE

Along with oil pulling, you need to maintain good dental hygiene. Brush your teeth daily after meals. Use non-fluoridated toothpaste. J.E. Phillips, D.D.S, the inventor of the Phillips Blotting Technique (see Chapter 1), recommends that you don't brush your teeth more than once a day. The reason for this is that too much brushing can be excessively abrasive. If you oil pull regularly, there is less of a need for brushing after *every* meal. Oil pulling for a few minutes at the end of the day is a good way to make sure all food particles are removed from your teeth before you go to bed.

Visit your dentist regularly to make sure your teeth are free of plaque and tarter and that there are no infections. If you oil pull regularly, you should not have any problems keeping your teeth in good shape.

When you first start to oil pull, your teeth may have some existing issues that need to be taken care of by a dentist, such as an abscessed tooth, unfilled cavity, or tarter which needs to be removed. In some people the hard calcium buildup that forms tarter may take a long time to dissolve. Having a dentist remove it will quickly relieve you of this problem and allow your gums to heal, as tarter causes chronic inflammation.

You also need to address other potential problems, such as amalgam fillings and root canals. Ideally, all metal should be removed from your mouth. If you must have metal, it should be gold or another metal with which you are compatible. If your goal is optimal health, amalgam fillings need to be replaced with composites and root canalled teeth need to be removed. However, as mentioned in Chapter 4, you need to study the issues involved and make the decision for yourself.

Major dental work can be expensive and traumatic. You may decide not to have additional work done or want to wait for the proper time. In these cases, you need to have some way to protect yourself from the toxins being emitted by your existing dental work. There are certain foods and nutrients that are effective in interacting with the heavy metals being released in your mouth. These items neutralize the harmful effects of the heavy metals or bind to them, preventing them from being absorbed by the body. The following section describes how to reduce your exposure to mercury and other heavy metals.

HEAVY METAL DETOXIFICATION
Follow the recommendations in this section if your mouth contains amalgam fillings or other heavy metals.

Trace Minerals
Trace minerals such as zinc and selenium are used in the construction of important enzymes that are necessary for hundreds of chemical reactions that are essential for good health and for life itself. When heavy metals like mercury and nickel are available, they can be used in place of the essential minerals in making these enzymes. This causes problems. When mercury is used in place of zinc, for instance, the resulting enzyme becomes dysfunctional. It is useless. The presence of too many of these dysfunctional enzymes hampers chemical processes in the body, which could lead to illness. If your diet is deficient in zinc and selenium or any other essential mineral, and heavy metals are available, these toxic minerals may take the place of the essential ones. To defend yourself from the effects of heavy metals, you can make sure you have ample amounts of the essential minerals available. This, in effect, dilutes the harmful affects of the heavy metals. With plenty of essential minerals available, fewer heavy metals have the opportunity of being used in the construction of enzymes.

If you have mercury or nickel in your mouth, you need to take a supplement that contains at least the minimum recommended dietary allowance of all the essential minerals. The RDA established by the US Committee on Dietary Allowances for zinc is 12 mg for adult women and 15 mg for adult men. For selenium it is 55 mcg for adult women and 70 mcg for adult men. You also need to take 2 mg of copper daily. Zinc and copper work together and must be taken together in a ratio of about eight-to-one. You could take twice the RDA of these minerals for added assurance that you are getting adequate protection. Too much zinc, selenium, and copper can become toxic too, so you don't want to overdo it. However, twice the RDA is well within the range of safety.

One mineral you don't want to take too much of is iron. Limit yourself to no more than the RDA, unless told otherwise by your physician.

A healthy diet will also contribute additional essential minerals, increasing your total daily intake above the recommended minimum.

Absorption of minerals from supplements and foods is greatly influenced by the diet. Vitamin C and dietary fat increase the release of essential minerals from foods during digestion and improve their rate of absorption. Low-fat diets can actually contribute to mineral deficiencies. If you eat a salad, for instance, using low-fat or no-fat dressing, you will only absorb a fraction of the minerals from the food. Adding a "good" source of fat can double, triple, and even quadruple the amount of minerals you absorb from the meal. A good source of fat could be from such things as avocado, nuts, cheese, olive oil, or coconut oil.

I recommend that you take at least 1,000 mg of vitamin C along with a multiple vitamin and mineral supplement containing at least the minimum daily requirement of zinc and selenium at the start of your day. Take the supplements with your breakfast and include a good source of fat to assure adequate absorption of the minerals.

Cilantro

Nature has provided us with numerous ways to treat disease and toxicity. Herbs have long been known for their healing properties. In recent years, one herb in particular has gained a reputation for its ability to chelate toxic heavy metals from the body. The herb is *Coriandrum sativum*, commonly known as cilantro, Chinese parsley, or coriander. Cilantro or Chinese parsley is the leafy portion of the plant, while coriander is the seed. It is the leafy portion of the plant that has gained the reputation as a natural chelating agent.

Cilantro is a member of the carrot family. It is commonly used for flavoring or garnishes in Asian and Mexican cooking.

The claim that cilantro is a powerful chelation agent is based on the research of Dr. Yoshiaki Omura, President and Founder of the International College of Acupuncture and Electro-Therapeutics, and Director of Medical Research of the Heart Disease Research Foundation, USA.

Dr. Omura found that antibiotics used to treat various infections were often ineffective in the presence of abnormal localized deposits of heavy metals like mercury, lead, and aluminum. Rigorous treatment with antibiotics and other drugs would calm symptoms for a time, but within a few months, the infections would recur. Careful examination of the patients revealed that the infections survived in localized areas of the body that were also areas of heavy metal accumulation. Heavy metal deposits co-existed with bacteria and viruses. He reasoned that the heavy metals somehow reduced the effectiveness of the medications, allowing the infections to continue. Heavy metal detoxification along with antibiotics were necessary in order to successfully treat these patients.

Cilantro's chelating properties were discovered almost by accident. In 1995 Dr. Omura found that patients who had eaten Vietnamese soup, which happened to contain cilantro, had an increased elimination of mercury in their urine. Further testing revealed that eating cilantro also increased urinary excretion of lead and aluminum. When cilantro was used with antibiotics, infections were eliminated for good. His research was recognized by other medical professionals and his findings published in peer-reviewed scientific journals.[13]

Approximately 1 tablespoon of cilantro, which is typical in food preparation, consumed daily over a three-week period was good enough to clear most of the heavy metal deposits from the body and allow the medications to do their job. Cilantro's cleansing effect wasn't limited to the digestive tract, but cleared heavy metals throughout the body, including the lungs, kidneys, endocrine organs, liver, and heart.

When dentists remove amalgam fillings, they take precautions to prevent the patient from ingesting or breathing mercury vapor and dust. A rubber dam is placed in the mouth with a strong air suction tube. Frequent water suctioning and washing is used to stop any mercury from going down the throat. Despite these precautions, mercury levels in the body normally rise after mercury removal. Dr. Omura demonstrated that if patients eat cilantro daily for two to three weeks after amalgam removal, mercury is effectively eliminated.[14] When exposed to large amounts of mercury, such as when amalgams fillings are removed, Dr. Omura recommends larger quantities of cilantro taken several times a day. In his studies on amalgams, Dr. Omura used powdered cilantro in 100 mg capsules taken four times daily.

Dr. Omura's studies on the chelating effects of cilantro have been independently confirmed by other researchers. Researchers at the Department of Atomic Energy in India have found that cilantro can also be used to purify contaminated water.[15] Cilantro acts as a filter, absorbing mercury from the water. Researchers report that cilantro was observed to remove inorganic and methylmercury from spiked ground water with "good efficiency."

Adding cilantro to your diet is an easy way to help protect yourself from mercury poisoning, especially if you have mercury amalgams. Cilantro is a pleasant tasting herb that can be used like parsley as a garnish and eaten whole to freshen the breath. It can also add flavor to Mexican or oriental dishes. It is popular in Indian cuisine. It can be used as part of the greens on sandwiches and in salads of all types.

Cilantro has the potential to mobilize more mercury from the tissues than the body can effectively eliminate. Bile, which is released into the digestive tract, is one of the major outlets for this mercury. Eating a high-fiber diet or taking chlorella supplements can help pull the mercury and other heavy metals out of the digestive tract.

Dietary Fiber

Dietary fiber is that portion of plant food that cannot be digested by human digestive enzymes. It passes in and out of the body mostly intact. Although fiber doesn't contribute much in the way of nutrients, it is invaluable in maintaining good digestive function. Dietary fiber has many other benefits, one of which is the ability to absorb toxins and heavy metals in the digestive tract and remove them from the body. Fiber also increases intestinal transit time, decreasing the risk of toxins being reabsorbed before they can be expelled. The foods highest in fiber are also among the healthiest—legumes, nuts, seeds, whole grains, vegetables, and fruits. Your diet should be rich in these foods.

Certain types of fiber are more effective than others at chelating or soaking up heavy metals and other toxins. There are two primary types of dietary fiber—soluble and insoluble. Pectin and guar gum, which are used as thickening agents in food processing, are examples soluble fiber. Insoluble fiber is the part of plant foods that we often call "roughage." Bran is an example of insoluble fiber. It is insoluble fiber that has the greatest chelating effect. The primary substance in the fiber that makes it an effective chelating agent is inositol hexaphosphate or simply IP6.

IP6 is an effective detoxifying agent and a potent antioxidant. Most of the research to date on IP6 has been on its ability to boost immune system function and fight cancer.[16-18] It has also been shown to be useful in preventing the formation of kidney stones.[19-20]

Whole grains, nuts, seeds, and legumes contain between 1-6 grams of IP6 per 100 gram (3.5 oz) serving. White flour products and polished white rice contain essentially no IP6 and are worthless as far as chelating heavy metals. Whole corn contains about 6 grams, sesame seeds 5 grams, whole wheat about 4 grams, and brown rice 2 grams each per 100 gram serving. IP6 is especially high in wheat and rice bran, with wheat bran containing nearly twice as much as rice bran. Abulkalam Shamsuddin, M.D., Ph.D., professor of pathology at the University of Maryland School of Medicine, known as one of the foremost authorities on IP6, recommends consuming 1-2 grams daily as a maintenance dose. You can get this amount from foods such whole grains, nuts, seeds, and legumes; from wheat and rice bran; or dietary supplements. One cup of cooked brown rice supplies about 2 grams of IP6. Adding a teaspoon or so of wheat bran to your meals can also supply the recommended amount.

Chlorella is a special fresh water algae that is used as a dietary supplement for the purpose of heavy metal detoxification. In many ways chlorella and bran are much alike. It is the fibrous portion of chlorella that attracts heavy metals and other toxins in the digestive tract and pulls them out of the body. Like IP6, chlorella is reported to boost the immune system and fight cancer. As with all sources of dietary fiber, digestive function is also benefited.

Chlorella is available in tablet, powder, and liquid form. The standard daily maintenance dose for adults is 3 grams or 30 ml of liquid extract. One teaspoon of powder contains 5 grams. You may want to start off slow by taking about half the recommend amount. Some people cannot tolerate chlorella and develop allergic-like symptoms such as difficulty breathing, chest pain, and hives. If that happens, discontinue use.

You can use a combination of dietary fiber, bran, IP6, and chlorella to help remove mercury from your body. Although you can, you need not use all of them. Eating foods with adequate dietary fiber is something that you should be doing all the time as part of a healthy diet. The supplements are just a bonus.

Don't eat a lot of IP6 rich foods or take IP6 or chlorella dietary supplements with your mineral supplements in the morning. The chelating effect of the IP6 and chlorella may reduce the amount of minerals you absorb. It is best to take IP6 or chlorella supplements just before or with lunch and dinner.

Antioxidants

Heavy metals can interfere with and damage many biological systems in the body. One of the major detrimental effects caused by mercury and other heavy metals is the creation of harmful free radicals. Mercury is highly toxic to living cells. It acts as a catalyst, transforming polyunsaturated fatty acids within cell membranes into free radicals. Consequently, the cell is damaged, dies, or mutates (i.e., becomes cancerous).

Once a free radical is formed, it randomly attacks neighboring molecules causing them to become free radicals as well. This process continues indefinitely, generating more and more free radicals. The greater the number of free radicals, the greater the damage they cause. Fortunately, we have a defense against these destructive terrorists—antioxidants. Antioxidants sacrifice themselves in the process of neutralizing free radicals. In this way, the antioxidants are used up. Antioxidants, therefore, must be replenished regularly to keep free radicals under control.

Where do we get antioxidants? From our food. Some of the most important antioxidant nutrients include vitamins A, C, E, lipoic acid, and CoQ10. Our bodies also use certain essential minerals such as zinc and selenium to make their own antioxidants. Vitamin C has been the primary antioxidant used to battle mercury intoxication. One of the reasons is that it can be taken in fairly large amounts without doing any harm. Mega doses of vitamin C are often administered intravenously to dental patients when they get their mercury amalgams removed. This helps greatly to prevent the toxic effects of mercury that finds its way into the bloodstream.

Most antioxidants are either water-soluble (vitamin C) or fat-soluble (vitamins A, E, CoQ10). Lipoic acid is unique in that it operates in a broader range of body tissues than other antioxidants, because it is both water- and fat-soluble. Its small size allows it to enter areas of the body not easily accessible to many other substances. For example, it can enter the cell nucleus and prevent free-radical damage to DNA. Lipoic acid works with vitamins C and E by regenerating their antioxidant potential after they have been exhausted by fighting free radicals. Unlike other antioxidants, lipoic acid also has a mild chelating effect.

You can never completely rid yourself of free radicals. They are constantly with us, being generated by various chemicals and toxins and even resulting from the normal processes of digestion and metabolism. Regardless of their origin, they are all damaging and need to be neutralized. As long as mercury is present in your body, it continues to generate free radicals and use up your antioxidant reserves.

If you have mercury amalgams, it is essential that you get adequate amounts of antioxidant nutrients in your diet. Your food alone may not supply enough to counter the destruction caused by the mercury in your mouth and that which may have collected in various parts of your body, such as your brain, liver, or kidneys. Dietary supplements are necessary.

The US RDA for vitamin A is 1,000 RE and for vitamin E it is 30 IU. Currently, there is no established recommended dose for lipoic acid. As a nutritional supplement, doses of 50 to 100 mg per day are generally recommended. As a therapeutic agent, higher doses may be used. You may find two types of lipoic acid being sold—R alpha-lipoic and S alpha-lipoic acids. The R form is derived from natural sources, while the S form is synthetic. The R form is about twice as effective as the synthetic.

If you are diabetic, check with your doctor before supplementing your diet with lipoic acid. Supplementation may reduce glucose and insulin levels, so you will have to monitor your sugar levels and adjust medication as needed.

MEDICATIONS
Drugs, Alcohol, and Tobacco

A number of drugs used to treat systemic diseases can cause oral complications ranging from xerostomic effects (drying of the mouth) to alterations in the surface structure of the enamel and mucous membranes. More than 400 over-the-counter and prescription drugs have xerostomic side effects including pain relievers (aspirin, ibuprofen), tricyclic antidepressants, antihistamines, and diuretics. Even body care products, such as antiperspirants, have a dehydrating effect that can greatly reduce salivary secretion. The antibiotic tetracycline can cause the incomplete or arrested development of tooth enamel when taken by a mother during pregnancy and by children during tooth development.

One popular drug associated with abnormal gum growth and development is cyclosporine, which is used as an immunosuppressant to prevent rejection of transplanted organs and bone marrow. It is also used as a treatment for type 2 diabetes, rheumatoid arthritis, psoriasis, multiple sclerosis, malaria, sarcoidosis, and several other autoimmune diseases. Other drugs that interfere with gum health include certain calcium ion channel blocking agents used in the treatment of various heart conditions and high blood pressure such as nifedipine and verapamil. The same is true of phenytoin, which is used in the treatment of epilepsy and also for the management of various neurological disorders.

Antibiotics and steroids often alter oral flora populations creating an environment that encourages fungal overgrowth in the mouth as well as the entire gastrointestinal tract. Hormone therapy can both encourage and discourage different types of oral flora, altering normal oral micro-populations.

Cancer patients are especially vulnerable to oral complications due to their lowered resistance to infection and to the effects of anti-cancer drugs and treatments. Chemotherapy drugs cause painful inflammation and ulcerations of the mucous membranes of the mouth and digestive tract, leaving tissues open to infection. Radiation therapy disrupts cell division in healthy tissue as well as in tumors, and affects the structure of the salivary glands and other tissues in the face and mouth. Oral complications are common after radiation therapy. A report on oral health and cancer therapy released by the U.S. Department of

Health and Human Services states, "Radiation can cause irreversible damage to the salivary glands, resulting in dramatic increase in dental caries." It goes on to say, "Oral mucosal alterations may become portals for invasion by pathogens, which may be *life-threatening* to immunosuppressed or bone-marrow-suppressed patients."[21]

Drugs can have a dramatic effect on our oral health. If at all possible it is best to avoid them. If drug therapy is necessary, it is even more important that you incorporate my entire Oil Pulling Therapy program to keep your immune system strong and harmful microbes under control.

Drugs with Dehydrating Effects

Analagesic mixtures	Cold medications
Anticonvulsants	Decongestants
Antiemetics	Diuretics
Antihistamines	Expectorants
Antihypertensives	Muscle relaxants
Antinauseants	Pain relievers
Anti-Parkinsonism agents	Psychotrophic drugs (CNS
Antiperspirants	depressants, tranquilizers)
Antispasmodic drugs	Sedatives
Appetite suppressants	

Drugs, alcohol, and tobacco all depress the immune system, allowing harmful bacteria to flourish. Alcohol and tobacco damage mucous membranes in the mouth, making it easier for bacteria to enter the bloodstream. It is best to avoid all alcoholic drinks, tobacco, and unnecessary drugs.

Many people find that as their health improves, the need for prescription drugs declines or becomes unnecessary. Obviously, if arthritic pain ceases, you no longer need to take pain-killers or anti-inflammatory drugs. Don't continue with the drugs simply out of habit. If there is no need for them, don't use them. Your progress will be quicker and more complete without them. If you are currently taking prescription drugs, monitor your progress as you work through the program, check with your doctor, and slowly wean yourself off the medications. Many people with crippling diseases, such as arthritis and diabetes, have been able to wean themselves completely off of drugs.

ACID/ALKALINE DYNAMICS

Your mouth can be acidic, alkaline, or even both. The mouth is a dynamic system where pH is constantly changing. At times it is acidic (low pH) at other times it may be alkaline (high pH). Different areas of the mouth often have varying levels of pH. Your mouth can literally be both acidic and alkaline at the same time.

Saliva pH can vary from about 5.0-8.0, although it more typically ranges between 6.0-7.4.[22] The pH range of saliva among those in ill health tends to be greater than among those in good health. A healthy mouth usually varies in pH by 0.4 or less. Those in ill health generally have a lower pH than those in good health. During the day, saliva pH is higher than at night. As we sleep, saliva secretion essentially stops.

Foods alter pH depending on their degree of acidity or alkalinity. Eating an orange, for example, would make the mouth more acidic. Carbohydrates affect pH by feeding acid-producing bacteria. Saliva buffers acids, increasing pH, but if blood sugar levels are high, saliva sugar levels can be high and feed bacteria. The pH on top of the tongue or around the molars may be lower than behind the front teeth, next to the salivary glands. After eating, pH often rises due to the buffering action of saliva, and then falls as bacteria feed on food particles and produce acids. It takes about an hour after eating for the pH to rise back up to normal levels. When we sleep, saliva secretion stops; without the buffering action of saliva, pH drops, so pH is lower during the night and in the morning when we awake than during the day.

The pH of your mouth is important because it determines whether teeth are being remineralized or demineralized. Minerals in your saliva crystallize, building up your teeth when the pH is relatively high (more alkaline) and demineralizes with it is low (more acidic), so your teeth are constantly being built up or broken down. The amount of time during which teeth are undergoing either the building phase or the demineralizing phase determines the strength of your teeth and your susceptibility to

151

tooth decay. Therefore, you want your saliva to have a higher pH (be more alkaline) most of the time.

Your eating habits greatly influence the acid/alkaline levels in your mouth. Carbohydrates in our diet supply the food that feeds mouth bacteria. This includes table sugar (sucrose), glucose, fructose, corn syrup, brown sugar, unrefined sugar, honey, molasses, and even starch, which is found in grains, vegetables, and fruits. After eating, bacteria will produce acids for approximately 30 minutes. If food particles get wedged in between teeth and folds in the skin, as they often do, bacteria can feed on it for hours, releasing acids the entire time. Keeping the mouth clean is an important step in preventing tooth decay and gum disease.

Sticky foods remain on teeth longer and present a greater risk than foods that are quickly cleared from the mouth. Caramels, gummy candies, and pastries are more of a threat than punch or juice, which may contain an equal amount of sugar. Refined flour products, including white bread, can be as bad as caramels. White bread, when chewed, becomes very sticky and clings to teeth. White bread, as well as donuts, pies, cookies, and such, can actually be more detrimental to your teeth than less-sticky candy.

Many parents give their children dried fruit such as fruit leather or raisins in the belief that they are healthy snacks. Dried fruit, however, is very sticky and is just as bad for the teeth as caramel candy.

Soda is bad as well. Although it doesn't cling to teeth like sticky candies and white flour products, it contains acids. These acids, like the acids formed by bacteria, can eat through tooth enamel and encourage the growth of acid-forming bacteria.

While supplemental vitamin C is recommended, chewable vitamin C is not. Vitamin C, also known as ascorbic acid, is highly acidic. In chewable form, vitamin C is strong enough to dissolve tooth enamel. An interesting study was done with chewable vitamin C.[23] Researchers dissolved a chewable tablet in distilled water and observed the effects the solution had on a healthy tooth. After four days in the solution the tooth began to decrease in size, and by the eighth day the surface of the tooth was so soft that it could be scraped away with a fingernail. When we eat sticky and acidic foods, acids continuously eat away at our teeth, making them soft and susceptible to decay.

If you eat acidic foods such as tomatoes, citrus fruits, and vinegar, you should have them with meals so they are diluted and flushed out of the mouth.

Raw vegetables do not stick to the teeth and require thorough chewing, which stimulates salivary flow. Increased saliva helps to clear food from the mouth and buffer acids. Adding more raw vegetables into the diet is an excellent way to offset cavity-promoting foods that may otherwise be eaten.

Several animal and human studies have shown that milk and dairy products have little potential for causing cavity development and may even protect against them.[24] Raw milk is especially good because it contains antibodies and enzymes that inhibit bacterial growth.[25] Although milk contains lactose, or "milk sugar," bacteria are not able to utilize it as easily as other forms of sugar. Dairy alkalizes the mouth, and with its high calcium and phosphorus content, contributes to the remineralization of the teeth.[26] Cheese is a powerful saliva stimulant, aiding in the removal of other foods and balancing pH and is, therefore, particularly effective in protecting teeth from decay. The anti-cavity potential of dairy is completely negated when sugar is added. Ice cream and sweetened yogurt, for instance, promote cavities rather than protect against them.

Nuts, especially if salted, are also effective in stimulating saliva flow and may help prevent cavities. Nuts are good sources of magnesium and trace minerals, which aid in bone and tooth formation. Because nuts are relatively hard, they are mildly abrasive, which helps clean the teeth. Some nuts, particularly cashews, contain chemicals that fight against the types of bacteria that cause tooth decay.[27]

Ever since Alexander Fleming discovered that penicillin killed bacteria in 1928 scientists have used fungal extracts as antibiotics. Mushrooms, likewise, contain antibacterial substances. Extracts from several varieties of editable mushrooms have been shown to inhibit the growth of S. mutans, the bacteria that is the primary cause of dental decay.[28] One of these is the shiitake mushroom, the most popular edible mushroom in Japan and widely popular elsewhere. Consuming shiitake mushrooms, and perhaps other mushrooms, may help protect against dental plaque and tooth decay.

At the end of a meal we often eat the wrong type of food—dessert! This leaves sugar in the mouth. It would be better to end meals by eating raw vegetables or dairy.

Drinking water after a meal or rinsing your mouth with water is also a good way to remove food particles and excess acids. You could also brush your teeth after every meal, but some dentists caution that too much brushing can be abrasive.

Sugar alcohols, such as xylitol, mannitol, and sorbitol, which are used as sugar substitutes, do not feed oral bacteria or promote tooth decay. Xylitol is of particular interest. Studies show that substitution of xylitol for sugar results in fewer cavities. The effect is greater than just the displacement of sugar; xylitol seems to have an anti-cavity effect. In one study, for instance, children who chewed xylitol-sweetened gum three times a day for two years developed fewer dental cavities than did their classmates who chewed nonxylitol gum. For this reason, products containing xylitol are often recommended as an aid against tooth decay.

Rinsing the mouth with a xylitol solution for a minute or two or chewing sugarless gum sweetened with xylitol is a good way to stimulate saliva and remove food particles. Xylitol is available in powder form at most good health food stores and online. To make your own xylitol "mouthwash," mix a little xylitol into a small amount of water and use as a rinse. If you like, you could even add a drop of mint extract to freshen your breath.

Rinsing the mouth with salt water can also be helpful. Salt stimulates salivary flow and has antiseptic properties. Salt has long been used as a food preservative because it inhibits bacteria growth. Salt on foods improves salivary flow, reducing the risk of developing cavities, as well as improving digestion. Sea salt is preferable over ordinary table salt because it contains many trace minerals that are beneficial to health.

Another factor that affects oral health is the frequency of food consumption. The more often you eat, the greater your risk of developing dental problems. Snacking between meals can be your worst enemy, especially if you snack on candy bars, chips, donuts, etc. Bacteria produce acid for about 30 minutes after exposure to sugar (if none of it sticks to the teeth). If a person eats three pieces of candy at one time,

Foods' Potential for Tooth Decay

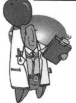

High Potential for Decay
Sugars and syrups
Candy
Pastries (cake, cookies, pie)
Frozen desserts (ice cream,
    popsicles)
Ready-to-eat breakfast cereals
Dried fruit
Chips, crackers, pretzels
Soft drinks (soda, punch)
Fruit juice
Canned fruit packed with syrup
Sweetened fruit
Sweetened beverages (eggnog,
    chocolate milk)
Jelly and jam
White flour products (bread,
    pasta, pancakes)
White rice

Moderate Potential for Decay
Cooked vegetables (except
    legumes)
Whole grains (wheat, corn, spelt,
    millet, brown rice, popcorn)
Hot Cereals (oats, cracked
    wheat)
Luncheon meats with added
    sugar
Whole grain pasta
Fruit

Low Potential for Decay
Raw vegetables
Legumes
Dairy
Meat, fish, poultry
Eggs
Fats and oils
Tea and coffee, unsweetened
Sugar substitutes (stevia,
    mannitol, sorbitol)

Potential to Prevent Decay
Cheese
Nuts
Shiitake mushrooms
Xylitol
Salt

the teeth would be exposed to about 30 minutes of acid demineralization. If that person were to eat the candy one piece at a time, one every half hour, the time of exposure to acid would increase to 90 minutes. The effect is three times as bad. Likewise, slowly sipping a soda between meals is much worse than drinking it with meals. Eating frequent small meals or continuously snacking or nibbling on carbohydrate-rich foods keeps acids in your mouth for extended periods of time, thus your teeth never have the opportunity to regain lost minerals.

It's best to avoid snacking between meals. If you must eat, snack on cheese, meat, eggs, nuts, raw vegetables, or something that is low-carb. Avoid sweets. Not only do they increase acid levels, they also reverse fluid flow within teeth, drawing acids and bacteria inside the teeth. If you do eat carbohydrates, drink water afterwards and rinse your mouth out or chew xylitol—sweetened gum. Even eating a little cheese or a few nuts will help counter the acid forming effects of the carbohydrates.

Avoid eating late at night or just before bedtime. Particles of food left in the mouth overnight will provide ample feeding for hungry bacteria. During the night, saliva production stops so the acid will not be buffered. Your mouth will be in an acidic state, demineralizing your teeth all night long.

DETOX PROGRAMS

If you follow the Oil Pulling Therapy program as outlined, you may begin to see improvements within days. Generally, minor problems show improvement within a few weeks. For chronic illnesses it may take several months or even a year or more. Some health problems may require more than oil pulling and dietary adjustments for complete healing to take place.

Years of accumulated toxins and tissue damage may require additional cleansing or other treatments to bring about complete recovery. Oil pulling is a very effective method of detoxification, and when combined with other methods of cleansing, can create a very powerful combination that is better than either one alone.

There are many types and methods of detoxification. Ready-made detox programs or products are available at most health food stores.

The most effective means of detoxification have been around for many years and have withstood the test of time. Most require little or no assistance. Traditional methods like fasting, juicing, sweat therapy (sauna), and the like are still considered the standard for cleansing and healing the body.

Describing each of the many methods of detoxification is beyond the scope of this book, but there are many books written on these topics. One of the best is my own book titled *The Detox Book: How to Detoxify Your Body to Improve Your Health, Stop Disease, and Reverse Aging.* This book provides step-by-step instructions for various methods of detoxification, including water fasting, juicing, oxygen therapy, exercise detoxification, heat therapy, colon cleansing, kidney cleansing, liver cleansing, herbal detoxification, and even mental/emotional cleansing. It provides details on dietary choices and explains how and why detoxification works. Another of my books that includes detox information is *Coconut Water for Health and Healing.* Among other things, this book describes the coconut water detox, a cleansing program that is in many ways superior to juice or water fasting. See the Bibliography for more information about these books.

OIL PULLING MAINTENANCE AND THERAPY
Maintenance

Oil pulling does not replace the need for brushing. You should continue to brush your teeth daily after eating. If you have no cavities or gum problems and are in good health, oil pulling once or twice a day may be all you need to maintain your health. Oil pulling should be done at least once a day in the morning before breakfast. It can be done twice; the best times are either just before lunch or in the evening sometime after dinner and before going to bed. Do not snack between oil pulling and going to sleep. You want to go to sleep with a clean, pH balanced mouth.

Therapeutic

If you have active gum disease, tooth decay, or any serious health problem, I recommend you follow the therapeutic protocol. Oil pull at least three times a day, once before each meal. Use what I call "medicated coconut oil." To make medicated coconut oil, add 1 drop of oregano or clove oil to every teaspoon of coconut oil. Oregano and clove oils have potent antimicrobial properties that will help kill mouth bacteria as well as viruses, fungi, and parasites. Clove oil is actually used as an oral disinfectant by dentists. The aroma you typically smell when you walk into a dental office comes from clove oil. You can use essential oils sold at most health food stores, or get them over the Internet. These oils are very strong and at full strength can irritate the skin. If you have a serious oral infection you may try using 2 drops for every 1 teaspoon of coconut oil.

Next, add the contents of one 30-50 mg gel capsule of CoQ10. It is difficult to open these gel capsules, so instead of trying to cut the capsule open, just put it in your mouth and crush it with your teeth. Suck out the contents and discard the gel cap shell. Follow by taking a spoonful of the coconut oil/oregano mixture.

CoQ10 topically applied to periodontal diseased gums has been shown to enhance healing.[29] Its antioxidant properties and its ability to improve energy production within the tissues both aid in the healing process.

Medicated Coconut Oil
1 teaspoon coconut oil
1-2 drops oregano or clove oil
1 30-50 mg CoQ10 gel capsule

Double or triple this recipe for oil pulling, depending on how much oil you typically use. Use the medicated coconut oil as long as you have an active infection in your mouth.

After brushing your teeth in the morning, rinse your mouth with a 3 percent hydrogen peroxide solution. Hydrogen peroxide is simply oxygenated water—water with an extra atom of oxygen. Hydrogen peroxide is used as a tooth whitener and disinfectant by dentists. Bacteria, viruses, and fungi can't tolerate too much oxygen. Even the tiny amount of extra oxygen in a 3 percent solution of hydrogen peroxide (97 percent water and 3 percent hydrogen peroxide) is enough to kill them. This makes hydrogen peroxide a very useful and safe antiseptic and an effective mouthwash. Hydrogen peroxide is more effective than commercial mouthwash and costs only a fraction of the amount. Rinse mouth with a 3 percent solution of hydrogen peroxide after brushing once a day, preferably in the morning, as this is the time when bacteria populations are at their highest.

When hydrogen peroxide comes into contact with germs, oxygen is released, causing the solution to bubble or foam. This is a sign it is killing germs. Since the mouth is full of germs, just a little will create foam in your mouth. Swish it around your mouth thoroughly and then spit it out. You can spit it into the sink as it is basically just water and dead germs.

If you have pain from a persistent infection, soak a cotton ball in hydrogen peroxide and place it inside the mouth next to the tooth. Keep the cotton ball in your mouth for 10 minutes. You can repeat this procedure two to three times a day until the pain subsides. Often the pain will go away after one day. If pain persists for more than three days, seek assistance from a dentist.

If you are having dental problems, it is important that you keep your mouth as clean as possible. Even when you are away from home you need to take care of your teeth. If you don't brush your teeth after a meal, then you should rinse your mouth with a xylitol solution or a mixture of baking soda and water to remove food particles and stabilize pH. If you don't have xylitol or baking soda solution, you can rinse your mouth with salt water.

Safety Factor

Oil pulling is completely harmless. All you are doing is putting vegetable oil, a food, into your mouth. You're not even going to swallow it. What could be more harmless than that? Women can do it during periods, pregnancy, and lactation. Regardless of ill heath or disease you can pull, unless there is some physical difficulty that prevents it. Oil pulling does not interact with any medications, so there are no contraindications. The only precaution is to be old enough to swish the oil in the mouth without swallowing. Generally, ages five and older can oil pull.

PROGRAM SUMMARY

Following Dr. Fife's Oil Pulling Therapy program, as outlined in this chapter, will enhance the cleansing effects of oil pulling and permenantly alter the microbial populations in your mouth in a positive way. Harmful or disease-causing bacteria will be reduced in favor of less troublesome bacteria, creating a healthy oral environment and enhancing your overall health. The main points of the program are summarized below. For details, refer to the discussion of each topic in the previous sections of this chapter.

Healthy Diet

Diet should consist primarily of fresh (and preferably organic) fruits, vegetables, meats, eggs, dairy, nuts and seeds, and whole grains. Avoid packaged, convenience foods and particularly refined grains and sweets. Avoid polyunsaturated and hydrogenated oils, sweets, and refined grains.

Supplemental Oil

Consume between 1-4 tablespoons of coconut oil daily. Use the oil in food preparation or take as a dietary supplement. Reduce or eliminate use of other vegetables oils.

Fluid Consumption

Drink one 12-ounce glass of water for every 25 pounds (12 kg) of body weight each day. It is best to drink pure, clean water without fluoride or chlorine.

Vitamins and Minerals

Take a multiple vitamin and mineral dietary supplement daily and include 500-1,000 mg of vitamin C. Limit supplemental calcium to 400-600 mg and match this with at least 400-600 mg of magnesium.

Dental Care

Brush and floss your teeth daily as needed. Visit the dentist for periodic check-ups. If you have existing root canals or amalgam fillings, take appropriate steps to resolve these issues to your satisfaction. If you have amalgam fillings, follow the daily mercury detox procedure below to reduce your exposure to mercury.

Mercury Detox (if you have amalgam fillings)

Trace Minerals

Take dietary supplements containing at least the RDA of zinc (15 mg), selenium (70 mcg), and copper (2 mg) daily. Zinc and copper need to be taken in a ratio of eight-to-one. Take mineral supplements in the morning with breakfast.

Cilantro

Eat 1 tablespoon fresh, chopped cilantro daily.

Dietary Fiber

Consume high-fiber foods including vegetables, nuts, seeds, and whole grains as a part of your daily diet. Supplement your diet with one of the following: 1-2 teaspoons of wheat bran, 1-2 grams IP6, or 3 grams chlorella. Take chelating supplements before or with lunch or dinner (do not take with mineral supplements at breakfast).

Antioxidants

Take a daily dietary supplement containing at least the RDA of vitamin A, vitamin E, lipoic acid, CoQ10, and a minimum of 1,000 mg of vitamin C. Take with mineral supplements at breakfast time.

Medications

Avoid all medications that are not absolutely necessary and all tobacco and alcohol products.

Maintaining Healthy pH

Be aware of the types of foods you eat and the effect they have on oral pH. Reduce or eliminate most sweets and refined grain products. Eat carbohydrates at mealtime. Avoid snacking between meals. If you do snack, eat foods with a low potential for tooth decay. After lunch and dinner, rinse your mouth with either xylitol solution, baking soda solution, or salt water. You can also use plain water if that is all you have available. You can also brush your teeth, but rinsing your mouth is more effective at controlling pH and removing food particles.

Detox Programs

Oil pulling can be combined with other forms of detoxification to enhance cleansing and healing, especially in the case of chronic, hard-to-treat conditions.

Maintenance and Therapy

For minor dental issues and daily maintenance, oil pull 1-2 times a day. To treat active dental and other health problems use medicated coconut oil and pull three times a day. If an infection is present in your mouth, rinse your mouth with 3 percent hydrogen peroxide solution after brushing your teeth in the morning.

YOUR SUCCESS

The level of success you achieve will depend on how closely you follow the program. If you don't experience the benefits you had hoped for, reevaluate how closely you are adhering to the program. The area where people tend to bend the rules the most is with their diet. It is easy to justify eating foods that don't support good health. Often we don't realize how much of this type of food we do eat.

I have purposely made the dietary recommendations very broad and simple, which can appeal to those with a wide range of personal beliefs and preferences. The main concept behind the food recommendations is to avoid those foods that have the most potential for negatively affecting health. That just happens to be processed, convenience foods—foods packaged in cans, bags, cartons, and plastic. With few exceptions, these foods are nutrient-deficient and loaded with questionable additives and incidental contaminants. Your diet is the single most important factor influencing your health. If you have health problems, chances are your diet is at least partially responsible.

Oil pulling is very powerful, and when combined with a sensible diet and other health-promoting activities, it can do wonders for your health. While oil pulling may not be the answer to every health problem, it has the potential to bring about remarkable improvement. It has the potential to allow the body to cure itself from numerous conditions, including so-called incurable ones.

You may notice changes almost immediately, or it may take some time. Improvements can be slow and subtle—so much so that you don't notice anything until one day you look back and say, "Hey, I didn't get the flu this year" or "My allergies didn't act up much this season." The most noticeable improvement will be to your oral health—fresher breath, healthier gums, and cleaner teeth. That, in itself, makes oil pulling worthwhile.

Note to Readers

Oil pulling is helping many people enjoy a better level of health. I would like to know how oil pulling is helping you. Please write and share your experiences with me. You can write to me in care of Piccadilly Books, Ltd., P.O. Box 25203, Colorado Springs, CO 80936, USA, or e-mail bruce@coconutresearchcenter.org. For more information about health and nutrition ask for a *free* copy/subscription to my *Healthy Ways Newsletter.* Subscriptions are only available via e-mail. To view a sample newsletter or to sign-up for a free subscription go to www.coconutresearchcenter.org/newsletter-sample.htm.

Myths and Misconceptions About Oil Pulling

The Internet is filled with explanations, theories, and procedures on why and how oil pulling works and the steps to take. Unfortunately, much of this information is wrong. Due to a severe lack of reliable information about oil pulling the Internet has been a major source of myths and misconceptions on the topic.

Keep in mind that anybody and anything can be posted on the Internet. It doesn't have to be true or accurate. The Internet is notorious for false information. Don't blindly believe anything you read. Be aware of the source of the information. If it is a research or academic institution or someone with notable credentials, the reliability is fairly high. If it is just someone's opinion, its accuracy may be questionable.

Because of the misinformation on the Web, I anticipate many people will have questions. I've devoted this section to answer some of these questions.

Q: Do I have to wait at least 1 hour after drinking water before I can oil pull?

A: Some sources claim you can't drink liquids any sooner than one hour before oil pulling. This is definitely wrong. It is actually better if you do drink some water just before pulling. This way you are properly hydrated and can produce the saliva needed for pulling. Often, people are dehydrated when they wake up in the morning. You need to get a drink to properly hydrate yourself before pulling.

Q: Do I have to wait at least four hours after eating before I can oil pull?

A: You can oil pull at any time. The reason for the recommendation to wait until food is digested is because pulling can cause the release of a lot of mucous. The mucous can disturb your stomach, causing nausea. For a beginner who is still not comfortable with putting oil in the mouth, it is best to wait at least an hour or two after eating. But for an experienced oil puller it isn't necessary.

Q: Must I only use sesame or sunflower oil for pulling?

A: No. These two oils are often recommended on the Internet but they are no better than any other oil and do not have the many health benefits associated with coconut oil, which I recommend.

Q: Does oil pulling draw toxins out of the bloodstream through blood vessels located in the mouth?

A: This is a popular explanation as to why oil pulling can detox the body, but it makes no sense. In order for toxins to be removed, they would have to come into direct contact with the oil. That means the oil would have to be absorbed through the mucous membranes and into the bloodstream. It would then have to grab the toxins and instantaneously jump back through the mucous membranes and back into the mouth before being carried off in the bloodstream. Even if the oil could go in and out of the bloodstream instantaneously, how is it going to tell which substances are toxic and should be removed and which ones are harmless and can be left alone? It can't. The way oil detoxifies is by absorbing bacteria and other organisms from the mouth, not the blood.

Q: Do I have to use a full tablespoon of oil?

A: No. Use whatever amount you feel comfortable with. A tablespoon is too much for many people. As you pull, your mouth will fill up even more as saliva is secreted. So you don't want to use too much oil.

Q: Some people have suggested that the healing effects of oil pulling are due to the essential fatty acids in the oil. Essential fatty acid deficient people absorb these fatty acids into the bloodstream through their mouths.

A: You will not absorb any appreciable amount of fatty acids by putting oil in your mouth for a few minutes and then spitting it out. The amount of oil you put into your mouth is the amount you will end up spitting out. Also, the essential fatty acid in sesame and sunflower oils is linoleic acid (omega 6). This fatty acid is available in almost all foods including meat, eggs, milk, vegetables, grains and all processed foods. An ordinary diet contains far more linoleic acid then what you would get from a tablespoon of sesame or sunflower oil. So the small amount in the oil used for pulling, will have absolutely no beneficial effect.

Q: Do I have to use cold-pressed or organic vegetable oils for pulling?

A: The belief that less refined oils are healthier than refined has led many websites to recommend cold-pressed or organic oils as the only option. Organic or cold pressed oil does not work any better than fully refined oils. Dr. Karach in his original talk recommended "refined" oil. Some websites that quote him have changed his words from "refined" to "cold-pressed" or "unrefined." You cannot take the quotes of Dr. Karach on the Internet at face value because his words have been altered on some of the websites. Also, others have unknowingly copied these altered texts and posted them on their own websites.

Q: Do I need to wait until the oil turns white before spitting it out?

A: The whiteness develops as thousands of tiny air bubbles are worked into the oil-saliva mixture. The oil will only turn white if you start with a very light colored or colorless oil. If you use an oil that is a deep yellow, like corn oil, or dark green, like olive oil, you will end up with a yellowish or greenish oil, not white. No matter how long and how hard you swish the oil in your mouth it will not turn white.

Q: Do I need to pull for a full 20 minutes?

A: That is like asking, "Do I need to brush all of my teeth?" If you brush your teeth for one minute, how thorough of a job will you do? Not very. The same is true with oil pulling. You need to give it adequate time, which is 15-20 minutes. However, if you are rushed and can only do it 5 or 10 minutes, that is better than not doing it at all.

Q: Must I focus my complete attention on my mouth the entire time I oil pull?

A: You need not sit in the lotus position and chant mantras while oil pulling. Some sources advocate doing nothing and focusing all your attention on your mouth while oil pulling. This is unnecessary. You can utilize your time more efficiently by doing other things at the same time. It makes the time go faster and the pulling more pleasant. While you pull, take your shower, prepare breakfast, go for a walk, read the paper, or work on the computer. You are more likely to stick with it if you can accomplish something useful at the same time. Then it will be easy to make oil pulling a part of your every day life and not a burden.

Q: Can oil pulling cure just about anything?

A: Oil pulling is not a cure. It is a means by which you remove germs from the mouth, relieving excessive stress on the immune system thus freeing the body to bring about improved health. This process can correct many health problems, but not all of them. It is unrealistic to believe oil pulling can and will cure everything. You shouldn't get discouraged if a certain health issue is not resolved. Its cause can be totally unrelated to oral health or immune function.

Q: Can I just hold the oil in my mouth and get the same results?

A: No. It's like sitting in a car with the engine turned off. You're in the car but you're not going anywhere. You need to start up the engine and get moving to accomplish anything. Likewise, you must work the oil in your mouth, pushing and pulling it through the teeth to draw bacteria out from between teeth and gums.

Q: Every time I start oil pulling I gag, what can I do?

A: This is fairly common for newcomers who don't like the taste or feel of oil in their mouths. In time, you get used to having oil in your mouth and the unpleasant feelings will decrease. In the meantime, if you start to gag, spit out the oil. Cough up any mucous in your throat, take a drink of water, and start over. You can also make the oil more tasteful by adding a couple of drops cinnamon or peppermint oil.

Q: Are there any medications that should not be used or that will interfere with oil pulling?

A: Oil pulling is completely harmless and does not interact with any drugs.

Q: Since oil pulling detoxifies the body, is it safe to do when pregnant or nursing?

A: Oil pulling reduces stress on the body by reducing bacteria load. This causes the body's immune system to become more efficient. The improved efficiency of the immune system actually improves fetal development and milk quality.

Q: Why haven't I seen the improvement that others report?

A: The biggest reason people don't see improvement is that they don't follow the program. For instance, they continue to eat junk foods, oil pull for only 5 minutes or less, don't pull every day, or don't drink enough fluids, and do things that do not promote improved health. You cannot expect improvement if you keep doing those things that destroy your health. Even if you do all the right things, you still need to allow time for it to work. Don't expect miracles to happen overnight. It may take many months or even years depending on your particular circumstances. Some health problems stem from causes unrelated to oral health or immune function. These may not fully respond to oil pulling therapy. Just because oil pulling may not "cure" a particular problem, however, doesn't mean it isn't useful. At the very least it will keep your mouth healthy and possibly prevent problems that may otherwise occur in the future.

Bibliography

Anonymous. *Phillips Blotting Technique*. Price-Pottenger Nutrition Foundation.

Breiner, M.A. *Whole Body Dentistry*. 1999. Quantum Health Press.

Bryson, C. *Fluoride Deception*. 2006. Seven Stories Press.

Cutler, A.H. *Amalgam Illness Diagnosis and Treatment: What You Can Do to Get Better, How Your Doctor Can Help*. 1999. Andrew Hall Cutler.

Fife, B. *Coconut Cures: Preventing and Treating Common Health Problems with Coconut*. 2005. Piccadilly Books, Ltd.

Fife, B. *The Coconut Oil Miracle, 4th Ed*. 2004. Avery Publishing.

Fife, B. *Coconut Water for Health and Healing*. 2008. Piccadilly Books, Ltd.

Fife, B. *The Detox Book: How to Detoxify Your Body to Improve Your Health, Stop Disease and Reverse Aging, 2nd Ed*. 2001. Piccadilly Books, Ltd.

Fife, B. *The Healing Crisis, 2nd Ed*. 2002. Piccadilly Books, Ltd.

Fife, B. *Virgin Coconut Oil: Nature's Miracle Medicine*. 2006. Piccadilly Books, Ltd.

Groves, B. *Fluoride: Drinking Ourselves to Death*. 2002. New Leaf.

Huggins, H. *It's All in Your Head: The Link Between Mercury Amalgams and Illness*. 1993. Avery Publishing.

Huggins, H. *Solving the MS Mystery: Help, Hope and Recovery*. 2002 Matrix, Inc.

Huggins, H. and Levy, T. *Uninformed Consent: The Hidden Dangers in Dental Care*. 1999. Hampton Roads Publishing Company.

Kulacz, R. and Levy, T.E. *The Roots of Disease: Connecting Dentistry and Medicine*. 2002. Xlibris Corp.

Price, W.A. *Dental Infections, Vol. 1 & 2*. 1923. Price-Pottenger Nutrition Foundation.

Price, W.A. *Nutrition and Physical Degeneration, 8th Ed*. 2008. Price-Pottenger Nutrition Foundation.

Stockton, S. *Beyond Amalgam: The Hidden Health Hazard Posed by Jawbone Cavitations, 2nd Ed*. 2000. Power of One Publishing.

Yiamouyiannis, J. *Fluoride the Aging Factor: How to Recognize and Avoid the Devastating Effects of Fluoride, 3rd Ed*. 1993. Health Action Press.

Ziff, S. *Silver Dental Fillings: The Toxic Time Bomb*. 1986. Aurora Press.

Books by Bruce Fife and Weston A. Price are available at your local health food store or bookstore. If you can't find them locally you can order them online from Piccadilly Books, Ltd. at www.piccadillybooks.com or from the Price-Pottenger Nutrition Foundation at www.ppnf.org.

References

Chapter 1: A New Approach to Better Health
1. Cromie, W.J. Discovering who lives in your mouth: Bacteria give clues to cancer and gum disease. *Harvard University Gazette*, August 22, 2002.

Chapter 2: Bacteria, Fungus, and Tooth Decay
1. Pihlstrom, B.L., et al. Periodontal diseases. *Lancet* 2005;366:1809-1820.

Chapter 3: All Disease Starts in the Mouth
1. Hughes, R.A. Focal infection revisited. *Br J Rheumatol* 1994;33:370-377.
2. Sconyers, J.R., et al. Relationship of bacteremia to tooth-brushing in patients with periodontitis. *J Am Dent Assoc* 1973;87;616-622.
3. Fine, D.H. and Stuchell, R. Correlation of levels of inflammation and inward particle penetration in human gingival. *J Dent Res* 1977;56:695-696.
4. Miller, W.D. The human mouth as a focus of infection. *Dent Cosmos* 1891;33:689-695.
5. Hunter, W. Oral sepsis as a cause of disease. *Lancet* 1900;i:215-216.
6. Hunter, W. The coming of age of oral sepsis. *Br Med J* 1921;i:859-861.

7. Billings, F. Chronic focal infections and their etiological relations to arthritis and nephritis. *Arch Int Med* 1912;9:484-498.

8. Rosenow, E.C. Focal infection and elective localization of bacteria in appendicitis, ulcer of the stomach, cholecystitis and pancreatitis. *Surg Gynecol Obsiet* 1921;33:19-26.

9. Mayo, C.H. Focal infection of dental origin. *Dental Cosmo* 1922;64:1206-1208.

10. US Department of Health and Human Services. Oral health in America: A report of the surgeon general. Rockville, MD:US Department of Health and Human Services, National Institute of Dental and Craniofacial Research, National Institutes of Health; 2000. Available at: http://www2.nidcr.nih.gov/sgr/sgrohweb/home.htm.

11. Eggleston, D.J. Teeth and infective endocarditis. *Aust Dent J* 1975;20:375-377.

12. Spaulding, C.R. and Friedman, J.M. subacute bacterial endocarditis secondary to dental infection. A case report. *NY J Med* 1975;41:292-294.

13. Kraut, R.A. and Hicks, J.L. Bacterial endocarditis of dental origin: report of a case. *J Oral Surg* 1976;34:1031-1034.

14. Kaplan, E.L. Prevention of bacterial endocarditis. *Circulation* 1977;56:139a-143a.

15. Oakley, C.M. Prevention of infective endocarditis. *Thorax* 1979;34:711-712.

16. Thornton, J.B. and Alves, J.C. Bacterial endocarditis. A retrospective study of cases admitted to the University of Alabama hospitals from 1969 to 1979. *Oral Sur Oral Med Oral Pathol* 1981;52:379-383.

17. Bayliss, R., et al. The teeth and infective endocarditis. *Br Heart J* 1983;50:506-512.

18. Siegman-Igra, Y., et al. Endocarditis caused by Actinobacillus actinomycetemcomitans. *Eur J Clin Microbiol* 1984;3:556-559.

19. Lieberman, M.B. A life-threatening, spontaneous, periodontitis-induced infective endocarditis. *J CA Dent Assoc* 1992;20:37-39.

20. Anonymous, Bad teeth and gums a risk factor for heart disease? *Harvard Heart Letter* 1998;9:6.

21. Millman, C. The route of all evil. *Men's Health* 1999;14:102.

22. DeStefano, F., et al. Dental disease and risk of coronary heart disease and mortality. *BMJ* 1993;306:688-691.

23. Muhlestein, J.B. Chronic infection and coronary artery disease. *Med Clin North Am* 2000;84:123.

24. Kozarov, E.V., et al. Detection of bacterial DNA in atheromatous plaques by quantitative PCR. *Microbes Infect* 2006;8:6887-693.

25. Kozarov, E.V., et al. Human atherosclerotic plaque contains viable invasive Actinobacillus actinomycetemcomitans and Porphyromonas gingivalis. *Arterioscler Thromb Vasc Biol* 2005;25:17-18.

26. Beck, J.D., et al. Periodontal disease and cardiovascular disease. *J Periodontal* 1996;67Suppl:1123-1137.

27. Carter, T.B., et al. Severe odontogenic infection associated with disseminated intravascular coagulation. *Gen Dent* 1992;40:428-431.

28. Currie, W.J. and Ho, V. An unexpected death associated with an acute dentoalveolar abscess—report of a case. *Br J Oral Maxillofac Surg* 1993;31:296-298.

29. Syrajanen, J., et al. Dental infections in association with cerebral infarction in young and middle-aged men. *J Intern Med* 1989;225:179-184.

30. Mattila, K.J., et al. Association between dental health and acute myocardial infarction. *BMJ* 1989;298:779-781.

31. Mattila, K.J., et al. Dental infections and coronary atherosclerosis. *Atherosclerosis* 1993;103:205-211.

32. Sikku, P., et al. Chronic Chlamydia pneumoniae infection as a risk factor for coronary heart disease in the Helsinki Heart Study. *Ann Intern Med* 1992;116:273-278.

33. Roivainen, M., et al. Infections, inflammation, and the risk of coronary heart disease. *Circulation* 2000;101:252-257.

34. Morer, G. Arthritis of the knee healed after dental avulsion. *Nouv Presse Med* 1975;4:2338.

35. Miller, W.D. The human mouth as a focus of infection. *Dent Cosmos* 1891;33:689-695.

36. Hunter, W. Oral sepsis as a cause of disease. *Lancet* 1900;i:215-216.

37. Billings, F. Chronic focal infections and their etiological relations to arthritis and nephritis. *Arch Int Med* 1912;9:484-498.

38. Billings, F. Chronic focal infection as a causative factor in chronic arthritis. *J Am Med Assoc* 1913;61:819-822.

39. Davidson, L.S.P., et al. Focal infection in rheumatoid arthritis. *Ann Rheum Dis* 1949;8:205-209.

173

40. Rashid, T. and Ebringer, A. Rheumatid arthritis is linked to Proteus—the evidence. *Clin Rheumatol* 2007;26:1036-1043.

41. Astrauskiene, D. and Bernotiene, E. New insights into bacterial persistence in reactive arthritis. *Clin Exp Rheumatol* 2007;25:470-479.

42. Kirdis, E., et al. Ribonucleotide reductase class III, an essential enzyme for the anaerobic growth of Staphylococcus aureus, is a virulence determinant in septic arthritis. *Microb Pathog* 2007:43:179-188.

43. Lens, J.W. and Beertsen, W. Injection of an antigen into the gingival and its effect on an experimentally induced inflammation in the knee joint of the mouse. *J Periodont Res* 1988;23:1-6.

44. Rubin, R., et al. Infected total hip replacement after dental procedures. *Oral Surg* 1976;41:18-23.

45. Schurman, D.J., et al. Infection in total knee joint replacement, secondary to tooth abscess. *West J Med* 1976;125:226-227.

46. Jacobsen, P.L. and Murray, W. Prophylactic coverage of dental patients with artificial joints: a retrospective analysis of thirty-three infections in hip prostheses. *Oral Surg* 1980;50:130-133.

47. Lindqvist, C., et al. Dental x-ray status of patients admitted for total hip replacement. *Proc Finn Dent Soc* 1989;85:211-215.

48. Newman, H.N. Focal sepsis—modern concepts. *J Irish Dent Assoc* 1986;14:53-63.

49. Scannapieco, F.A., et al. Oral bacteria and respiratory infection: effects on respiratory pathogen adhesion and epithelial cell proinflammatory cytokine production. *Annals of Periodontology* 2001;6:78-86.

50. Latronica, R.J. and Shukes, R. Septic emboli and pulmonary abscess secondary to odontogenic infection. *J Oral Surg* 1973;31:844-847.

51. Rams, T.E. and Slots, J. Systemic manifestations of oral infections. In: *Contemporary Oral Microbiology and Immunology*. Slots J., Taubaman, M.A. editors. St. Louis: Mosby, 1992;500-510.

52. Loesche, W.J., et al. A possible role for salivary bacteria in aspiration pneumonia. *J Dent Res* 1995;74:127.

53. Von Mutius, E. Of attraction and rejection—asthma and the microbial world. *N Engl J Med* 2007;357:1545-1547.

54. Kraft, M., et al. Mycoplasma pneumoniae and Chlamydia pneumoniae in asthma: effect of clarithromycin. *Chest* 2002;121:1782-1788.

55. Gibbs, R.S., et al. A review of premature birth and subclinical infection. *Am J Obstet Gynecol* 1992;166:1515-1528.

56. Offenbacher, S., et al. Actinobacillus actinomycetemcomitans infection associated with low birth weight. *J Dent Res* 1993;72:2157.

57. Offenbacher, S., et al. Periodontal infection as a risk factor for preterm low birth weight. *J Periodont* 1996;67(10 Suppl):1103-1113.

58. Moliterno, L.F., et al. Association between periodontitis and low birth weight: a case-control study. *J Clin Periodontol* 2005;32:886-890.

59. Krejci, C.B. and Bissada, N.F. Women's health issues and their relationship to periodontitis. *J Am Dent Assoc* 2002;133:323-329.

60. Leon, R., et al. Detection of Porphyromonas gingivlis in the amniotic fluid in pregnant women with a diagnosis of threatened premature labor. *J Periodontol* 2007;78:1249-1255.

61. Herrera, J.A., et al. Periodontal disease severity is related to high levels of C-reactive protein in pre-eclampsia. *J Hypertens* 2007;25:1459-1464.

62. Mapstone, N.P., et al. Identification of Helicobacter pylori DNA in the mouth and stomachs of patients with gastritis using PCR. *J Clin Pathol* 1993;46:540-543.

63. Nguyen, A.M., et al. Detection of Helicobacter pylori in dental plaque by reverse transcription-polymerase chain reaction. *J Clin Microbiol* 1993;31:783-787.

64. Van Dyke, T.E., et al. Potential role of microorganisms isolated from periodontal lesions in the pathogenesis of inflammatory bowel disease. *Infect Immun* 1986;53:671-677.

65. Dickinson, C.J. Mouth bacteria as the cause of Paget's disease of bone. *Med Hypotheses* 1999;52:209-212.

66. Yoshihara, A. et al. A longitudinal study of the relationship between periodontal disease and bone mineral density in community-dwelling older adults. *J Clin Periodontol* 2004;31:680-684.

67. Lerner, U.H. Inflammation-induced bone remodeling in periodontal disease and the influence of post-menopausal osteoporosis. *J Dent Res* 2006;85:596-607.

68. Ebisu, S. and Noiri, Y. Oral biofilms and bone resorption. *Clin Calcium* 2007;17:179-184.

69. Nishimura, F., et al. Periodontal disease and diabetes mellitus: the role of tumor necrosis factor-alpha in a 2-way relationship. *J Periodontol* 2003;74:97-102.

70. Mealey, B.L. and Rethman, M.P. Periodontal disease and diabetes mellitus. Bidirectional relationship. *Dent Today* 2003;22:107-113.

71. Mealey, B.L. and Oates, T.W. diabetes mellitus and periodontal diseases. *J Periodontol* 2006;77:1289-1303.

72. Engebretson, S., et al. Plasma levels of tumour necrosis factor-alpha in patients with chronic periodontitis and type 2 diabetes. *J Clin Periodontol* 2007;34:18-24.

73. Grossi, S.G. Treatment of periodontal disease and control of diabetes: an assessment of the evidence and need for future research. *Ann Periodontol* 2001;6:138-145.

74. Lacopino, A.M. Periodontitis and diabetes interrelationships: role of inflammation. *Ann Periodontol* 2001;6:125-137.

75. Pucher, J and Stewart, J. Periodontal disease and diabetes mellitus. *Curr Diab Rep* 2004;4:46-50.

76. Aldous, J.A., et al. Brain abscess of odontogenic origin: A case report. *J Am Dent Assoc* 1987;115:861-863.

77. Marks, P.V., et al. Multiple brain abscesses secondary to dental caries and severe periodontal disease. *Br J Oral Maxillofac Surg* 1988;26:244-247.

78. Andrews, M. and Franham, S. Brain abscess secondary to dental infection. *Gen Dent* 1990;38:224-225.

79. Hedstrom, S.A., et al. Chronic meningitis in patients with dental infections. *Scand J Infect Dis* 1980;12:117-1121.

80. Zachariades, N., et al. Cerebral abscess and meningitis complicated by residual mandibular ankylosis. A study of the routs that spread the infection. *J Oral Med* 1986;41:14-20.

81. Fernando, I.N. and Phipps, J.S.K. Dangers of an uncomplicated tooth extraction. A case of Streptococcus sanguis meningitis. *Br Dent J* 1988;165:220.

82. Perna, E., et al. Actinomycotic granuloma of the gasserian ganglion with primary site in a dental root. A case report. *J Neurosurg* 1981;54:553-555.

83. Barrett, A.P. and Buckley, D.J. Selective anaesthesias of peripheral branches of the trigeminal nerve due to odontogenic infection. *Oral Surg* 1986;62:226-228.

84. Kim, J.M., et al. Dental health, nutritional status and recent-onset dementia in a Korean community population. *Int J Geriatr Psychiatry* 2007; 22:850-855.

85. Nakayama, Y, et al. Oral health conditions in patients with Parkinson's disease. *J Epidemiol* 2004;14:143-150.

86. McGrother, C.W., et al. Multiple sclerosis, dental caries and fillings: a case study. *Br Dent J* 1999;187:261-264.

87. Stein, P.S., et al. Tooth loss, dementia and neuropathology in the Nun study. *J Am Dent Assoc* 2007;138:1314-1322.

88. Zigangirova, N.A. and Gintsburg, A.L. Molecular approach for development of new medicaments for chronic infections treatment. *Zh Mikrobiol Epidemiol Immunobiol* 2007;(4):103-109.

89. Crippin, J.S. and Wong, K.K. An unrecognized etiology for pyogenic hepatic abscesses in normal hosts: dental disease. *Am J Gastroenterol* 1992;7:1740-1743.

90. Kshirsagar, A.V., et al. Periodontal disease is associated with renal insufficiency in the Atherosclerosis Risk in Communities (ARIC) study. *Am J Kidney Dis* 2005;45:650-657.

91. Pollmacher, T., et al. Influence of host defense activation on sleep in humans. *Adv Neuroimmunol* 1995;5:155-169.

92. Kirch, W. and Duhrsen, U. Erythema nodosum of dental origin. *Clin Invest* 1992;70:1073-1078.

93. Smith, A.G., et al. Fulminant odontogenic sinusitis. *Ear Nose Throat J* 1979;58:411-412.

94. Miller, E.H. and Kasselbaum, D.K. Managing periorbital space abscess. Secondary to dentoalveolar abscess. *J Am Dent Assoc* 1995;126:469-472.

95. Ishak, M.A., et al. Endogenous endophthalmitis caused by Actinobacillus actinomycetemcomitans. *Can J Ophthalmol* 1986;21:284-286.

96. Bieniek, K.W. and Riedel, H.H. Bacterial foci in the teeth, oral cavity, and jaw—secondary effects (remote action) of bacterial colonies with respect to bacteriospermia and subfertility in males. *Andrologia* 1993;25:159-162.

97. Shelley, W.B. Urticaria of nine year's duration cleared following dental extraction. *Arch Derm* 1969;100:324-325.

98. Russi, E.W., et al. Septic pulmonary embolism due to periodontal disease in a patient with hereditary hemorrhagic telangiectasia. *Respiration* 1996;63:117-119.

99. Suzuki, J., et al. A fatal case of acute mediastinitis caused by periodontal infection. *Nihon Kyobu Shikkan Gakkai Zasshi* 1992;30:1847-1851.

100. Marks, P.V, et al. Multiple brain abscesses secondary to dental caries and severe periodontal disease. *Br J Oral Maxillofac Surg* 1988;26:244-247.

101. Losli, E. and Lindsey, R. Fatal systemic disease from dental sepsis. *Oral Surg Oral Med Oral Pathol* 1963;16:366-372.

102. Gallagher, D.M., et al. Fatal brain abscess following periodontal therapy: a case report. *Mount Sinai J Med* 1981;48:158-160.

103. Palank, E.A., et al. Fatal acute bacterial myocarditis after dentoalveolar abscess. *Am J Cardiol* 1979;43:1238-1241.

Chapter 4: Deadly Dentistry

1. Berlin, M.H., et al. On the site and mechanism of mercury vapor resorption in the lung. *Archives of Environmental Health* 1969;18:42-50.

2. Kudak, F.N. Absorption of mercury from the respiratory tract in man. *Acta Pharmacology Toxicology* 1965;23:250-258.

3. Svare, C.W., et al. The effect of dental amalgams on mercury levels in expired air. *Journal of Dental Research* 1981;60:1668-1671.

4. Reinhardt, J.W., et al. Mercury vapor expired after restorative treatment: preliminary study. *Journal of Dental Research* 1979;58:2005.

5. Ziff, S. *The Toxic Time Bomb*. Santa Fe, NM; Aurora Press, 1986.

6. Svare, C.W., et al. The effect of dental amalgams on mercury levels in expired air. *Journal of Dental Research* 1981;60:1668-1671.

7. Heintze, V, et al. Methylation of mercury from dental amalgam and mercuric chloride by oral streptococci in vitro. *Scandinavian Journal of Dental Research* 1983;91:150-152.

8. Huggins, H. *It's All In Your Head: The Link Between Mercury Amalgams and Illness*. Garden City Park, NY:Avery Publishing, 1993.

9. Gosselin, R.E., et al. *Clinical Toxicology of Commercial Products,* *5th Ed.* Philadelphia, PA:William & Walkins, 1984.

10. Fagin, D. Second thoughts about fluoride. *Scientific American* January 2008.

11. Skolnick, A. New doubts about benefits of sodium fluoride. *JAMA* 1990;263:1752-1753.

12. Riggs, B.L., et al. Effect of fluoride treatment on the fracture rate in postmenopausal women with osteoporosis. *N Engl J Med* 1990;322:802-809.

13. Lee, L. Fluoride alert. *To Your Health* October 2004.

14. US Department of Agriculture. A*ir Pollutants Affecting the Performance of Domestic Animals. Agricultural Handbook No. 380.* Revised. 1972, p. 109.

15. Weinstein, L.H. Effects of Fluorides on Plants and Plant Communities: An Overview. In: Shupe JL, Peterson HB, Leone NC, (Eds). *Fluorides: Effects on Vegetation, Animals, and Humans.* Salt Lake City, Utah: Paragon Press, 1983, pp. 53-59.

16. Janet Raloff, The St. Regis Syndrome. *Science News* July 19, 1980, pp. 42-43.

17. Fagin, D. Second thoughts about fluoride. *Scientific American* January 2008.

18. Nelsons, D.G.A., et al. Crystallographic structure of enamel surfaces treated with topical fluoride agents: TEM and XRD considerations. *J Dent Res* 1984;63:6-12.

19. Jin, Y. and Yip, II. Supragingival calculus: formation and control. *Crit Rev Oral Biol Med* 2002;13:426-441.

Chapter 5: The Miracle of Oil Pulling

1. Amith, H.V., et al. Effect of oil pulling on plaque and gingivitis. *JOHCD* 2007;1:12-18.

2. Tritten, C.B. and Armitage, G.C. Comparison of a sonic and a manual toothbrush for efficacy in supragingival plaque removal and reduction of gingivitis. *J Clin Periodontol* 1996;23:641-648.

3. Asokan, S., et al. Effect of oil pulling on Streptococcus mutans count in plaque and saliva using Dentocult SM Strip mutans test: A randomized, controlled, triple-blind study. *J Indian Soc Pedod Prevent Dent* 2008;26:12-17.

4. Anand, T. D., et al. Effect of oil-pulling on dental caries causing bacteria. *African Journal of Microbiology Research* 2008;2:63-66.
5. Asokan, S., et al. Effect of oil pulling on *Streptococcus mutans* count in plaque and saliva using Dentocult SM Strip mutans test: A randomized, controlled, triple-blind study. *JISPPD* 2008;26:12-17.

Chapter 6: Oil Pulling Basic Training
1. Roberts, G.J., et al. Dental bacteraemia in children. *Pediatr Cardiol* 1997;18:24-27.
2. Slanetz, L.W. and Brown, E.A. Studies on the numbers of bacteria in the mouth and their reduction by the use of oral antiseptics. *J Dent Res* 1949;28:313-323.

Chapter 7: Dr. Fife's Oil Pulling Therapy
1. Price, W.A., *Nutrition and Physical Degeneration, 8th edition*. La Mesa, CA:Price-Pottenger Nutrition Foundation, 2008.
2. Carroll, K.K. and Khor, H.T. Effects of level and type of dietary fat on incidence of mammary tumors induced in female Sprague-Dawley rats by 7,12-dimethylbenz()anthracene. *Lipids* 1971;6:415-420.
3. Reddy, B.S. and Maeura, Y. Tumor promotion by dietary fat in azoxymethane-induced colon carcinogenesis in female F344 rats: influence of amount and source of dietary fat. *J Natl Cancer Inst* 1984;72:745-750.
4. Cohen, L.A. and Thompson, D.O. The influence of dietary medium chain triglycerides on rat mammary tumor development. *Lipids* 1987;22:455-461.
5. Cohen, L.A., et al Influence of dietary medium-chain triglycerides on the development of N-Methylnitrosourea-induced rat mammary tumor. Can*cer Res* 1984;44:5023-5028.
6. Mascioli, E.A., et al. Medium chain triglycerides and structured lipids as unique nonglucose energy sources in hyperalimentation. *Lipids* 1987;22:421-423.
7. Fife, B. *Coconut Cures: Preventing and Treating Common Health Problems with Coconut*. Colorado Springs, CO: Piccadilly Books, Ltd., 2005.
8. Ershow, A.G., et al. Intake of tapwater and total water by pregnant and lactating women. *Am J Public Health* 1991;81:328-334.

9. Dauteman, K.W., et al. Plasma specific gravity for identifying hypovolaemia. *J Diarrhoeal Dis Res* 1995;13:33-38.

10. Fife, B. *Coconut Water for Health and Healing.* Piccadilly Books, Ltd., 2008.

11. Leggott, P.J., et al. The effect of controlled ascorbic acid depletion and supplementation on periodontal health. *Journal of Periodontology* 1986;57:480-485.

12. Abraham, G.E. and Grewal, H. Effect on the mineral density of calcaneous bone in postmenopausal women on hormonal therapy. *J Reprod Med* 1990;35:503-507.

13. Omura, Y. and Beckman, S.L. Role of mercury (Hg) in resistant infections and effective treatment of Chlamydia trachomatis and Herpes family viral infections (and potential treatment for cancer) by removing localized Hg deposits with Chinese parsley and delivering effective antibiotics using various drug uptake enhancement methods. *Acupunct Electrother Res* 1995;20:195-229.

14. Omura, Y., et al. Significant mercury deposits in internal organs following the removal of dental amalgam, & development of pre-cancer on the gingiva and the sides of the tongue and their represented organs as a result of inadvertent exposure to strong curing light (used to solidify synthetic dental filling material) & effective treatment: a clinical case report, along with organ representation areas for each tooth. *Acupunct Electrother Res* 1996;21:133-160.

15. Karunasagar, D. et al. Removal and preconcentration of inorganic and methyl mercury from aqueous media using a sorbent prepared from the plant Coriandrum sativum. *J Hazard Mater* 2005;118:133-139.

16. Vucenik, I., et al. Comparison of pure inositol hexaphosphate and high-bran diet in the prevention of DMBA-induced rat mammary carcinogenesis. *Nutrition and Cancer* 1997;28:7-13.

17. Ullah, A. and Shamsuddin, A.M. Dose-dependent inhibition of large intestinal cancer by inositol hexaphosphate in F344 rats. *Carcinogenesis* 1990;11:2219-2222.

18. Singh, R.P., et al. Inositol hexaphosphate inhibits growth, and induces G1 arrest and apoptotic death of prostate carcinoma DU145 cells: modulation of CDKI-CDK-cyclin and pRb-related protein-E2F complexes. *Carcinogenesis* 2003;24:555-563.

19. Grases, F., et al. A new procedure to evaluate the inhibitory capacity of calcium oxalate crystallization in whole urine. *International Urology & Nephrology* 1995;27:653-661.

20. Ohkawa, T., et al. Rice bran treatment for patients with hypercalciuric stones: experimental and clinical studies. *Journal of Urology* 1984;132:1140-1145.

21. http://www2.nidcr.nih.gov/sgr/sgrohweb/chap5.htm.

22. Guyton, A.C. *Textbook of Medical Physiology, 8th Ed.* Philadelphia, PA:W.B. Saunders Company, 1991.

23. Giunta, J.L. Dental erosion resulting from chewable vitamin C tablets. *Journal of the American Dental Association* 1983;107:253-256.

24. Rugg-Gunn, A.J., et al. The effect of different meal patterns upon plaque pH in human subjects. *British Dental Journal* 1975;139:351-356.

25. Effert, F.M. and Gurner, B.W. Reaction of human and early milk antibodies with oral streptococci. *Infect Immun* 1984;44:660-64.

26. McDougall W. Effect of milk on enamel demineralization and remineralization in vitro. *Caries Res* 1977;11:166-72.

27. Weber, C. Eliminate infection (abscess) in teeth with cashew nuts. *Medical Hypotheses* 2005;65:1200.

28. Shouji, N., et al. Anticaries effect of a component from shiitake (an edible mushroom). *Caries Res* 2000;34:94-98.

29. Hanioka, T., et al. Effect of topical application of coenzyme Q10 on adult periodontitis. *Mol Aspects Med* 1994;15 Suppl:S241-248.

Index

183

About the Author

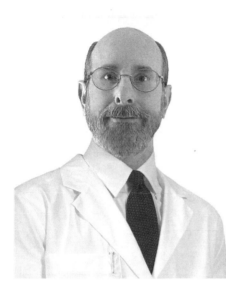

Bruce Fife, C.N., N.D.

Dr. Bruce Fife, C.N., N.D., is an author, speaker, certified nutritionist, and naturopathic physician. He has written over 20 books including *Coconut Water for Health and Healing*, *The Coconut Oil Miracle* and *Eat Fat, Look Thin*. He is the publisher and editor of the *Healthy Ways Newsletter* and serves as the president of the Coconut Research Center (www.coconutresearchcenter.org), a non-profit organization whose purpose is to educate the public about the health and nutritional aspects of coconut.

Dr. Fife is recognized internationally as the foremost authority on the health and nutritional aspects of coconut and related topics. Dr. Fife was the first one to gather together the medical research on the health benefits of coconut oil and present it in an understandable and readable format for the general public. As such, he travels throughout the world educating medical professionals and laypeople alike on the wonders of coconut. For this reason, he is often referred to as the "Coconut Guru" and many respectfully call him "Dr. Coconut."

To view a sample copy of Dr. Fife's *Healthy Ways Newsletter* or to sign-up for a free subscription go to www.coconutresearchcenter.org/newsletter-sample.htm.

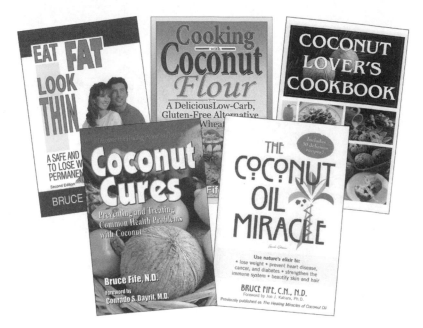

The Coconut Oil Miracle, 4ᵗʰ Edition*

This is the book that started the coconut oil revolution. Originally published in 2000 this book was the first to reveal the health benefits of coconut oil to the public. It uncovers the politics behind the coconut oil smear campaign sponsored by competing industries and how science brought it back into popularity. In this book you will learn why coconut oil is considered the healthiest oil on earth and how it can protect you from heart disease, diabetes, influenza, herpes, candida, and even HIV.

*Formerly titled *The Healing Miracles of Coconut Oil*

Coconut Cures:
Preventing and Treating Common Health Problems with Coconut

This book reveals the health benefits of the entire coconut—the oil, meat, milk, and water. Discusses in detail why coconut protects against heart disease. Includes an A to Z resource section explaining how to use coconut to treat specific health problems.

Eat Fat, Look Thin:
A Safe and Natural Way to Lose Weight Permanently

This book explains how to use coconut oil to lose excess weight, stimulate metabolism, increase energy, and improve thyroid function. Many people have been able to reduce or even completely eliminate thyroid medication by following the recommendations in this book.

Coconut Water for Health and Healing

Coconut water is a refreshing beverage that comes from coconuts. It's a powerhouse of nutrition containing a complex blend of vitamins, minerals, amino acids, carbohydrates, antioxidants, enzymes, health enhancing growth hormones, and other phytonutrients. It's unique nutritional profile gives it the power to balance body chemistry, ward off disease, fight cancer, and retard aging.

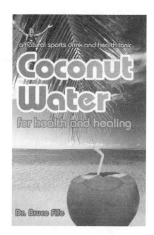

Coconut Lover's Cookbook

This book contains 450 recipes using coconut oil, meat, milk, and cream. Recipes include a variety of beverages, salads, soups and stews, curries, main dishes, side dishes, and desserts. Explains how to use coconut oil for cooking and how to get the recommended amount of coconut oil into your diet.

Cooking with Coconut Flour:
A Delicious Low-Carb, Gluten-Free Alternative to Wheat

Coconut flour is made from finely ground coconut meat. It is very high in health promoting dietary fiber and contains no gluten. Coconut flour can be used to make delicious tasting gluten-free breads, cakes, cookies, muffins, and other baked goods. Coconut flour can improve digestion, help regulate blood sugar, protect against diabetes, help prevent heart disease and cancer, and aid in weight loss.

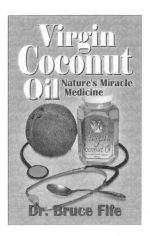

Virgin Coconut Oil:
Nature's Miracle Medicine

A short overview on the health aspects of virgin coconut oil with numerous case histories and testimonials. Discover how people are successfully using virgin coconut oil to prevent and treat high cholesterol, high blood pressure, arthritis, fibromyalgia, candida, herpes, allergies, psoriasis, influenza, diabetes, and much more.

 Piccadilly Books, Ltd.
www.piccadillybooks.com

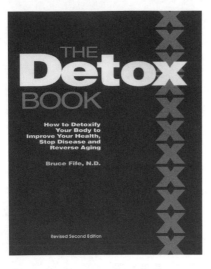

The Detox Book:
How to Detoxify Your Body to Improve Your Health, Stop Disease, and Reverse Aging

We live in a toxic world. People today are exposed to chemicals in far greater concentrations than were previous generations. Thousands of tons of man-made chemicals and industrial pollutants are poured into our environment and our food supply daily. As a consequence, we are getting sick. In no other time in the history of the world has degenerative disease been as prominent as it is today. Diseases that were rare or unheard of a century ago are now raging like a plague. Nature, however, has provided us with the solution. Our bodies are amazingly resilient. If the disease-causing toxins are removed, the body will heal itself. This book outlines the steps you need to take to thoroughly detoxify and cleanse your body from these disease-causing agents. You will also learn how to reduce your toxic exposure and how to strengthen your immune system.

The Healing Crisis

Natural health treatments that focus on removing disease-causing influences using the body's own power of healing often brings on an unpleasant reaction known as the *healing crisis*. In this book you will learn how to distinguish between a healing crisis and a disease crisis (illness or allergy). You will learn how healing works, what to do and what not to do to facilitate healing, and how to cope with unpleasant symptoms until the crisis is over. If you undergo any type of natural healing program, you must be well informed about the symptoms and processes of the healing crisis. This book will guide you through the natural healing process.

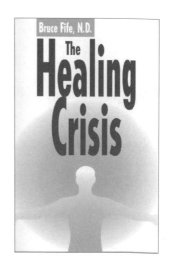

 Piccadilly Books, Ltd.